CRAFTING A CLONING POLICY

CRAFTING A CLONING POLICY
From Dolly to Stem Cells

ANDREA L. BONNICKSEN

Georgetown University Press / Washington, D.C.

Georgetown University Press, Washington, D.C. 20007
© 2002 by Georgetown University Press. All rights reserved.

Printed in the United States of America

10 9 8 7 6 5 4 3 2 1
2002

This volume is printed on acid-free, offset book paper.

Library of Congress Cataloging-in-Publication Data

Bonnicksen, Andrea L.
    Crafting a cloning policy : from Dolly to stem cells / Andrea L. Bonnicksen.
    p. cm.
    Includes bibliogorapical references and index.
    ISBN 0-87840-370-1 (cloth : alk. paper)—ISBN 0-87840-371-X (pbk. : alk.
    paper)
        1. Cloning—Government policy—United States. I. Title.

    QH442.2 .B66 2002
    174′.966065—dc21

                                                        2002020865

In memory of
Hans and Oline Bonnicksen
and
Anton and Lena Dahl

CONTENTS

LIST OF TABLES

ACKNOWLEDGMENTS

The early research for this book was done while I was on sabbatical leave from Northern Illinois University. I owe special thanks to the generosity of the Center for Biomedical Ethics at the University of Virginia, with Jonathan D. Moreno as its director and John Fletcher as its former director. My stay there as a visiting scholar in fall 1999 opened up the excellent facilities at the university to me and enabled me to participate in activities with the Center's associates. I also owe thanks to Albert R. Jonsen, former director of the Department of Medical History at the University of Washington, for enabling a visiting scholar affiliation at that university in spring 2000. For helping me to understand the nature of Food and Drug Administration oversight, I thank Philip D. Noguchi, Suzanne L. Epstein, and Malcolm Moos, Jr., of the Center for Biologics Evaluation and Research. I am also grateful to Robert H. Blank for his insightful suggestions and to Marlene Sokolon, Genevieve Dame, and Kim Dubose for their research help.

ABBREVIATIONS

ART	assisted reproductive technology
AS	adult stem
ASRM	American Society for Reproductive Medicine
BIO	Biotechnology Industry Organization
CA-SLHERA	Committee on Appropriations, Subcommittee on Labor, Health and Human Services, and Education, and Related Agencies (U.S. Senate)
CBER	Center for Biologics Evaluation and Research
CLHS-SPHS	Committee on Labor and Human Resources, Subcommittee on Public Health and Safety (U.S. Senate)
CS-ST	Committee on Science, Subcommittee on Technology (U.S. House)
DHEW	U.S. Department of Health, Education and Welfare
DHHS	U.S. Department of Health and Human Services
EAB	Ethics Advisory Board
EG	embryonic germ
EGE	European Group on Ethics in Science and New Technologies
ES	embryonic stem
FDA	Food and Drug Administration
FDCA	*Food, Drug, and Cosmetic Act of 1938*
HERP	Human Embryo Research Panel
HFE Act	*Human Fertilisation and Embryology Act of 1990*
HFEA	Human Fertilisation and Embryology Authority
HGAC	Human Genetics Advisory Committee
HGC	Human Genetics Commission
IDHL	*International Digest of Health Legislation*
IGM	inheritable genetic modification
IND	investigational new drug application
IRB	institutional review board
IVF	in vitro fertilization
NBAC	National Bioethics Advisory Commission
NCB	Nuffield Council on Bioethics
NDA	new drug application
NIH	National Institutes of Health
PCB	President's Council on Bioethics
PHSA	*Public Health Service Act*
RAC	Recombinant DNA Advisory Committee
SCNT	somatic cell nuclear transfer

CHAPTER 1

INTRODUCTION

In mid-1996, a lamb, Dolly, was born in Scotland after having been cloned from a mammary gland cell of an adult female sheep. The announcement of Dolly's birth in early 1997 provoked an unusually intense international reaction that combined alarm about the potential for human cloning with fascination for the lamb gazing from her pen at milling crowds of reporters and photographers. Her birth quickly became part of the popular culture and the grist for whimsical musings. "Mary had a little lamb," one poetic couple wrote, "she cloned it from a ewe. The lamb, confused, [did ask] the sheep. Am I me or you?" (Seares and Seares 1997). Headlines along the lines of "Hello Dolly," "Bring in the Clones," "Clone on the Range," and "There Can Never Be Another Ewe" masked unsettling feelings about what it would be like to clone human beings. A technique thought to be impossible and long the topic of fiction had been accomplished, pending replication of the study.

Dolly's birth was achieved through somatic cell nuclear transfer (SCNT), in which technicians transferred a body (somatic) cell from an adult sheep to an enucleated egg and prompted it to begin dividing as an embryo (Wilmut et al. 1997). The embryo was then transferred to a surrogate ewe for gestation and birth, and the resulting lamb, Dolly, had the same genome as the sheep that was the source of the somatic cell. The birth turned out to be a harbinger of other unusual discoveries announced from research institutes in the United Kingdom, Australia, and other nations in well-attended press conferences. Ian Wilmut and colleagues in the United Kingdom celebrated the birth of Polly the lamb, who was cloned from fetal cells and genetically engineered. Downgrading the attention over Dolly's birth, the scientists who had enabled the births of both Dolly and Polly stated that Dolly had been a "mere detour" and "just the gilt on the gingerbread" to the road to Polly, the real star (Klotzko 1998, 131; Wilmut, Campbell, and Tudge 2000, 182). Polly was engineered to have a human gene in her cells that would enable her to produce a protein in her milk to treat hemophilia. Nuclear transfer to facilitate the production of transgenic animals signaled the commercial cloning possibilities for animal biotechnology (Pennisi 1997). Then, in 2000, researchers in Oregon announced the first birth of a primate, a rhesus monkey, who had the gene of another species in her body cells. To produce the monkey, researchers inserted a DNA sequence controlling for the green fluorescent protein of a glowing jellyfish into a primate egg, fertilized it, and then transferred it to a surrogate rhesus monkey (Chan et al. 2000; Vogel 2001c). The resulting infant, ANDi ("inserted DNA" spelled backward), carried the gene in all her cells, although the gene did not express.

The isolation and culture of human embryonic stem (ES) cells in 1998 piqued immediate interest as scientists predicted that SCNT could be used to create tailor-made genetically compatible cells and tissues for human medical therapies. These and other discoveries demonstrated that SCNT was only one cog in a set of intersecting techniques in which, as Wilmut, Campbell, and Tudge (2000, 9) put it, inheritable genetic modifications (IGMs) were the "conceptual leader" and cloning was the vehicle to enable the modifications.

While these events occupied the attention of ethicists and scientists, cloning cyclically attracted the attention of policymakers. Cloning emerged as a political issue when, on two separate occasions, scientists announced they would try to clone humans, and it ebbed when observers persuaded themselves that the cloning technology was too primitive to succeed with humans in the near future and that minimum controls in place would deter scientists from the attempt. Yet cloning is only one part of a mix of rapidly changing reproductive and genetic technologies. Novel prospects of genetic manipulations, spurred by the anticipated completion of the human genome project, have provoked Lee Silver and others to write of the newly emerging "reprogenetics" and an advisory body in Canada to write about reproductive and genetic technologies (RGTs) (Silver 1997, 9; Parens and Juengst 2001). Whatever its moniker, the expected convergence of these technologies contributes to a sense of urgency to develop plans for managing intersecting technologies that have heretofore been discussed primarily on a technique-by-technique basis.

Despite continued concerns in the United States and elsewhere about the prospect of human cloning, no new laws on cloning had emerged in the United States by the end of 2001. Still, several states had enacted anticloning laws, the House of Representatives passed a broad bill making human SCNT a criminal act, and the Senate held more hearings on cloning. Efforts to outlaw reproductive SCNT, whether successful or not, are noteworthy because never before in the quarter-century history of assisted reproductive technologies (ARTs) has Congress seriously tried to restrict a technique designed to enable conception, and especially not preemptively to bar a category of biomedical research still hypothetical for humans.

The absence of new cloning legislation by the end of 2001 is in some ways curious, given widespread uneasiness about cloning and the singular nature of the technique. Yet, in other ways, the quick enactment of a new law is not surprising. Congress has traditionally not limited scientific studies and medical research, and the potential commercial and public health benefits of research that fall short of human reproductive cloning leave legislators wary of casting too wide a restrictive net. Moreover, constitutional liberty protections that embrace free inquiry and reproductive privacy place a high burden on those aiming to bar scientific and medical procedures. This burden would have been a difficult obstacle to overcome in 1997 for a hypothetical technique that had successfully produced only one mammal. In addition, lingering disagreements about embryo research have complicated legislative initiatives. To clone, one would first need to create an embryo through nuclear transfer. Concerns about creating and destroying human embryos have superimposed the unresolved politics of embryo research onto the politics of cloning.

The cloning issue, with the public skepticism it produces, creates a sense of mission to take clear action, which would most efficiently take the form of a single anticloning law passed by Congress. Yet, it is not clear that such a law will be passed or that, if enacted, it would be appropriate or even effective. If narrowly crafted, it might meet the immediate goal of preventing the transfer of an embryo created through SCNT to a woman's uterus within the United States. But the difficulties of crafting legislation with the right degree of precision are weighty, and judicial challenges to a proscriptive law would leave the issue unsettled for some time. More important, an anticloning law, tailored for one specific technique, would not provide a framework for the parade of innovative reproductive and genetic technologies certain to emerge in the years to come.

For these and other reasons, it makes sense to look at broadly defined policy rather than narrowly defined law to consider what realistic and appropriate responses might best be crafted in a time when cloning is no longer a far-fetched possibility. Policy is a broad concept that refers to norms and principles that guide behavior and contribute to a general framework for making decisions. A policy, as described by Daniel Callahan (1990, 160), "does not map out in advance the exact choice to be made in each situation," but instead "affirm[s] . . . a given cluster of values and goals" that will in turn guide individual choices. A policy is more than a list of rules or a simple prohibition; it includes a vision and a method for carrying out that vision. Policy derived from statutes, administrative codes, and recommendations by government-sponsored advisory bodies can be thought of as public policy. Policy developed in the private sector, which includes clinical practices, recommendations by privately sponsored advisory bodies, and guidance documents from professional associations, can be thought of as private policy. If one looks solely to the law, one may emerge with a crimped notion of constraints on behavior. If one looks to policy, one may emerge with a more robust notion of guiding principles and expectations.

An editorial in the journal *Nature* chided U.S. policymakers by pointing out that while cloning "marches on" in animal biotechnology, the "world's scientific superpower has so far failed to deliver a satisfying contract between researchers and citizens at large on this issue" (*Nature* 1998). If one looks for a newly crafted law to assess the accuracy of this observation, it does indeed seem that a contract has not yet been reached. Yet, if one seeks the foundations of a cloning policy that are pieced together, however inelegantly, from existing policy resources, the accuracy of the observation is less obvious. What are the key features of cloning policy in the United States? More significantly, what do these features show about the country's readiness to manage problematic reproductive and genetic technologies in the future?

This book uses reproductive cloning as a case study to inform efforts to develop a responsible policy structure for managing innovative future technologies. It assumes a degree of vitality of policy resources that can be overlooked when attention turns to the inchoate public policy governing ARTs in the twenty-plus years since Louise Brown was born through the use of in vitro fertilization (IVF). It assumes, in other words, that policy resources look stronger when examined together through the eye of one who is looking for their potential than when they are studied in isolation.

This book focuses on the type of reproductive cloning used to create Dolly—reproductive SCNT. I use "reproductive cloning" interchangeably with reproductive SCNT when reports, hearings, and other sources indicate that cloning technologies other than SCNT are at issue. Yet, as technologies advance, "cloning" falls behind in its ability to discriminate among procedures and uses. Moreover, this simple term does not distinguish among sources of nuclei for transfer, which include undifferentiated embryo cells and differentiated fetal and adult cells. Embryo cell, fetal somatic cell, and adult SCNT, all of which have been performed in animals, are variations of cloning that would raise distinct ethical issues if attempted in human procreation (Bonnicksen 1997).

Using reproductive SCNT as a case study to take stock of today's policy inventory makes sense for at least two reasons. First, Dolly's birth elicited unusually intense responses. This is, after all, a technique that arguably shifts the nature of procreation. As one law professor contended, "cloning is replication, not reproduction, and represents a difference in kind not in degree in the manner in which human beings reproduce" (U.S. Senate, Committee on Labor and Human Resources, Subcommittee on Public Health and Safety [CLHS-SPHS] 1997a). Here, a person could arrange the genetic makeup of his or her child by selecting a person to donate a body cell and, with it, that person's genome. No new mingling of genes would be needed, although the child would differ in many ways from the person whose body cell was used for the conception. With imaginative uses, parents in different locations and at different times could give birth to spaced genetic twins or triplets who share the genome of a person the parents found worthy enough to repeat and could challenge the nature of social and biological relationships. The very oddity—some would say repugnance—of the procedure has elicited a high degree of interest and a sense that reproductive cloning is a matter of relevance to all humans (Kass 1997).

Second, despite a widespread feeling that cloning should not be allowed, efforts to prevent cloning revealed the practical difficulties of regulating a scientific technique. Fewer than two years after Dolly's announced birth, researchers reported that they had isolated human ES cells. They lauded human ES cells as "universal" cells with great promise for medical therapies, particularly to produce cells and tissues for transplantation. One envisioned form of ES cell therapy was to use cloning technology to create ES cell lines that would be compatible with the intended recipient. Thus, the ES cell controversy injected a new and important distinction into the concept of cloning. Now the same technique of SCNT theoretically could promote two separate ends: producing a child (reproductive SCNT) and treating patients (therapeutic SCNT). It could be used for an end deemed troubling to some (to create a cloned child) and beneficent to others (to treat persons with diseases and conditions). Barring the one could inadvertently foreclose the other. Cloning is a study of the pragmatic challenges of monitoring techniques that do not fit into neat categories.

Although reproductive cloning presents an intriguing lens for evaluating the policy readiness of the United States for managing innovative reproductive technologies, writing a book about this technique brings risks. Any number of events can occur between the day a laser printer ejects the manuscript's final pages and the day the completed book arrives. If scientists prematurely attempt to use reproductive SCNT to create a human and the effort leads to an unsafe pregnancy, a neonatal death, or an infant with disorders, reproductive cloning would effectively be shut down for years to come. In contrast, if an apparently healthy infant is born through reproductive SCNT, this would defuse some of the controversy and open the door to a new set of policy options and ethical issues about how to integrate cloning into the clinical setting.

Unpredictable events can also take place in Congress, where members continue to introduce and even vote on bills. The executive and legislative branches have been at odds over the issue and the ES cell issue became an unexpected litmus test for President George W. Bush's administration. All this makes it hard to predict what will happen. By the end of 2001, numerous cloning bills and ES cell bills were being considered in Congress and hearings were in process. Even if a law targeting SCNT is passed in Congress, this will not be the final answer. For one thing, a law of this unusual nature would likely be challenged and the denouement may be a long time in coming. In addition, as one legal scholar has noted, law is too easily perceived as the "end of discussion," when in fact it is the beginning of— a "repository for"—discussion (Jabbari 1990, 40). A prohibitive law would be as likely to raise as to answer questions and the politics of the event would be unlikely to fade into oblivion. Moreover, reproductive SCNT may be practiced in other nations, which will keep it alive as an issue and continue the need to weigh policy options in light of international collaborative research and the movement of people conceived through the technique from one nation to another.

To cushion against unpredictable contingencies, this book focuses on a bounded period of time—1997 to 2000, the years immediately after Dolly's announced birth. Although scientific and political events have continued unabated since 2000 and will be mentioned as appropriate, policy activities from 1997 to 2000 provide a useful window for viewing policy resources. During these three years, efforts to enact a cloning law revealed deep-seated conflicting values and dividing lines that would be unlikely to change appreciably in the years to come. Then, with ES cell discoveries and the recognition that SCNT was part of a tapestry of interrelated techniques, the need to make careful policy distinctions grew in importance. The ES cell issue also shifted embryo research from the narrow world of infertility treatment to the mainstream world of therapeutic medicine. In so doing it mobilized an active political constituency sensitive to limits on medical research.

The years between 1997 and 2000 also showed that reproductive SCNT was serious business in animal biotechnology. First, Wilmut and colleagues verified in 1998 that Dolly had in fact been created through reproductive SCNT (Solter 1998). Other research teams replicated the feat with modified procedures to four other species: mice, cows, goats, and pigs. Investigators at the University of Hawaii reported the birth of Cumulina the mouse, who had been cloned from the cumulus cells that surround the egg, and the births of other mice who were not only clones, but clones of clones (Wakayama et al. 1998). Several research groups in Japan reported the births of female calves cloned from oviductal and cumulus cells (Normile 1998). In 1999, a bull was cloned from the skin cells of another bull. In 2000, five pigs named Millie, Christa, Alexis, Carrel, and Dotcom, were cloned from somatic cells (Polejaeva et al. 2000; *Seattle Times* 2000).

These births demonstrated that reproductive SCNT could be used for different species and with diverse cells in the body—not just cells connected with the female reproductive system. The growing number of births suggested that cloning could become efficient and perhaps safe. Early evidence indicated that cloned animals might be born aged, with cells that had shorter than normal telomeres (ends of chromosomes that shorten with each cell division) (Shiels et al. 1999). Later studies, however, showed that on the contrary, cloned calves might have longer than normal telomeres and therefore have longer life spans (Lanza et al. 2000). Cumulina, the first mouse cloned by reproductive SCNT, died in 2000 at the age of two years, seven months, which is seven months older than the average mouse life span (*Nature* 2000). Dolly continued to be healthy, although overweight and arthritic, and she mated with the ram David to give birth to a daughter lamb, Bonnie. Enough animals had been cloned for scientists to observe that animals were less similar to one another in physiology and temperament than expected (Wilmut, Campbell, and Tudge 2000, viii, 5, 10).

Despite some assurances about reproductive SCNT, the procedure still was clearly not safe. Maladies were reported among cloned animals, including hypoplasia in calves (Renard et al. 1999), larger than normal fetuses among calves conceived by fetal cell and embryo cell nuclear transfer (Pennisi and Vogel 2000, 1724), longer than normal gestation, and a high rate of fetal and neonatal deaths (Wilmut, Campbell, and Tudge 2000, 293). Researchers involved with cattle cloning estimated that one in seven calves cloned by SCNT has potentially fatal complications such as abnormal lung development

(Vogel 2001b, 809). The larger than normal fetal size may have contributed to limb deformities and other problems by constricting the ability of the fetuses to move in the uterus during gestation (Talbot 2001, 45).

If reservations about reproductive SCNT pervaded political debates between 1997 and 2000 and if legislators introduced numerous bills to Congress, why did Congress fail to enact an anticloning law? Why, as one journalist put it, when "much of the world seems to have instinctively condemned the idea of cloning people [is] this country [the United States] struggling to find a way to just say no?" (S. Cohen 1997, 14). To set the stage for this query, chapter 2 proposes three features of American political culture that partly explain the lack of an early and instant policy response to reproductive cloning: technological optimism, residual conflicts over human embryo research, and the private policy tradition in research and development relating to ARTs. These and other aspects of the political culture set a deliberate pace for policy development and offer guidance about politically realistic policy options. The chapter also distinguishes among four policy approaches to managing reproductive SCNT: (1) legislation with narrow arc, (2) legislation with broad arc, (3) existing regulatory mechanisms, and (4) regulatory mechanisms with adjustments. This sets the stage for chapters 3, 4, and 5, which examine efforts by Congress to enact a law, either narrowly or broadly crafted, and chapters 6, 7, and 8, which examine some of the existing regulatory mechanisms and potential adjustments to them.

Chapter 3 focuses on the early responses to reproductive SCNT in 1997 and the crafting of legislative options. In that year members of Congress introduced bills to restrict reproductive cloning and convened hearings to debate its ethical and policy implications. President Bill Clinton asked the National Bioethics Advisory Commission (NBAC) to issue a report on the ethics of cloning, and the commission held a series of open meetings to deliberate about the ethics of cloning and to make policy recommendations. Diverse views about the moral status of the human embryo emerged as markers in the legislative alternatives, and they rendered an anticloning law elusive.

The year 1998 began with Richard Seed, a physicist, announcing his intention to clone a human being. Although Seed's announcement seemed more an act of self-aggrandizement than a serious effort to clone, the scenario spurred members of Congress to introduce more detailed bills. Senate sponsors of an anticloning bill attempted to by-pass the usual procedures and bring the bill directly to the Senate floor without committee hearings. The move prompted accelerated lobbying by a growing constituency of scientific and medical groups that felt threatened by broadly crafted anticloning bills and began to contest the pro-life and other groups that favored laws restricting research into reproductive cloning. Chapter 4 traces these and other congressional developments in 1998 that reinforced the rudiments of the politics of cloning.

After the Senate voted down the 1998 attempt to bypass committee hearings, reproductive cloning moved to the back stage, a rerun of what occurred after the NBAC issued its report in 1997. Then, in late 1998, the isolation of human ES cells elevated reproductive cloning issues to the policy agenda again, with the potential use of SCNT for therapy rather than reproduction. Chapter 5 reviews the political activities of 1999 when Congress and the NBAC again convened experts, this time to understand the science of stem cells and to identify ethical and legal issues associated with research using ES cells. This set the stage for heated divisions that have not yet reached their crescendo.

Chapters 6, 7, and 8 address existing regulatory mechanisms and their role in a cloning policy. Periodically during the 1997–2000 period, the Food and Drug Administration (FDA) asserted that it had regulatory authority over cloning. If legislation is elusive or not fully effective, what role might the FDA play in policy development? Chapter 6 examines this question, keeping in mind that FDA oversight would be a central feature of an approach relying on existing mechanisms.

Both the president and Congress agreed between 1997 and 2000 that no federal funds would be used to clone a human being. Although federal funding of human reproductive SCNT is an extremely remote possibility, the government may eventually fund subsidiary research that touches on therapeutic SCNT or expanded ES cell research and, in the process, mobilizes a long-standing policy apparatus that has traditionally not been used for reproductive technologies. President Bush opened a narrow door to funding of ES cell research in 2001, which for the first time brought federal oversight to research involving human embryos, however narrowly defined. This activates another component of existing mechanisms. Chapter 7 explores the role federal research protections might play in a reproductive cloning policy.

Wilmut and colleagues have observed that people "tend to object as a matter of course to any new, exotic technology that affects the human body." The innate suspicion eventually levels out, they write, and sometimes the "technology that once seemed outlandish, or even diabolical, is widely accepted as normal practice" (Wilmut, Campbell, and Tudge 2000, 273–74). Similarly, Lori Andrews quotes two fertility specialists who, writing over thirty years ago, suggested that for new reproductive technologies, people pass through stages of "horrified negation" to "negation without horror" to "slow and gradual curiosity" to "finally a very slow but steady acceptance" (quoted in Kolata 1997c). It is not unreasonable to suppose that a moderation of attitudes toward reproductive SCNT will eventually take place. In fact, reports stating that reproductive SCNT is unethical "at this time" leave open the possibility of a re-examination after (and if) the technique is determined to be safe in animal biotechnology. Although serious safety issues preclude human reproductive SCNT in the immediate future (Jaenisch and Wilmut 2001), it is not necessarily an endorsement of the technique to think prospectively about what policy apparatus would govern the integration of reproductive SCNT into society if its safety were assured. Chapter 8 first reviews state involvement thus far, which has taken the form of anticloning laws. It then explores the potential policy role state legislatures and courts may play if reproductive SCNT or its variations were ever practiced.

Shared expectations relating to reproductive cloning can be identified in national and international protocols, reports, and laws. While the policies of other nations are not legally binding on the United States, they suggest policy options and norms that can guide policy formation. Chapter 9 first compares policy approaches of three nations similar to the United States—the United Kingdom, Australia, and Canada—with an eye to this question: How might policy practices in these nations inform policy development in the United States? To provide a more global context to the cloning issue, chapter 9 also reviews laws enacted in other countries and international agreements that touch upon innovative reproductive technologies.

Chapter 10 returns to the four policy approaches and looks with favor to a model that would adjust and refine existing regulatory mechanisms. Of all the approaches, this has the greatest potential for setting the stage for the complex intersection of technologies in the future. The chapter uses the key features of cloning policy to date to ask what issues remain in the construction of a policy for managing innovative technologies in the years to come.

Cloning has risen and fallen as a policy issue since 2000. In 2001, Panos Zavos, a reproductive physiologist in the United States; Severino Antinori, an infertility specialist in Italy; and Avi Ben-Abraham, an Israeli physician, announced they would attempt to clone a human being by 2003 in an unnamed country, possibly a country in the Middle East (Vogel 2001b; Pickrell 2001). Also in 2001, scientists affiliated with Clonaid, an organization dedicated to human cloning, announced they were devoting resources to attempting reproductive SCNT. Clonaid was founded by Claude Vorilon from Montreal, who goes by the name Rael, and the organization's creed revolves around its leader's alleged visit to a spaceship. Using funds contributed by potential clients, Clonaid had fifty women ready to act as surrogates for embryos created through cloning, and an anonymous couple who wish to be the first to have a child through reproductive SCNT (Talbot 2001). This couple was fertile, and the intention of the wife and husband was to bring a child into the world who shared the genome of their baby who had died at ten months of age. One hundred couples were on Clonaid's waiting list; most were on the list because of infertility.

Members of Congress held hearings and introduced bills in 2001, only this time the hearings featured witnesses, such as Raelian Brigitte Boisselier (of Clonaid), who claimed the merits of cloning, as well as Rudolph Jaenisch and other critics who reiterated the dangers associated with animal cloning (U.S. House, Committee on Energy and Commerce, Subcommittee on Oversight and Investigations 2001). Despite Raelian efforts to keep the location of their laboratory secret, FDA regulators found and inspected the laboratory, after which Boisselier signed an agreement not to try reproductive SCNT on U.S. soil. She did not pledge to refrain from trying it elsewhere (*New York Times* 2001).

On the ES cell issue, President Bush spent several months considering whether to approve funding of ES cell research. On August 9, 2001, he announced in a nationally televised speech that he would approve federal funding of sixty-four existing ES cell lines under carefully controlled conditions, and that he would create the President's

Council on Bioethics (PCB) to monitor ES cell research and to recommend guidelines. With each resurrection of the cloning issue and with each new twist of the ES cell issue, the intersection of scientific techniques became that much more complex. An understanding of the events between 1997 and 2000 directs attention to resources for a cloning policy that can be marshaled in anticipation of intersecting reproductive and genetic technologies still on the horizon.

CHAPTER 2

Underpinnings of Policy Development

Restive energy brewed on the heels of Dolly's announced birth. One common response was astonishment of the sort one might expect when a central dogma of biology—that body cells were irreversibly specialized—lay demolished. Reporters converged on the Roslin Institute where the birth had taken place. In the weeks after the announced birth, the investigators took over 2,000 telephone calls and gave interviews to more than one hundred reporters. Sixteen film crews with fifty photographers arrived to take pictures of Dolly. The coverage across the world was, as Ian Wilmut put it, "of all possible hues: sober, thoughtful, pompous, portentous, shrill, frivolous, whimsical, and just plain daft" (Wilmut, Campbell, and Tudge 2000, 221–22).

Energy also coalesced among observers and policymakers who geared up to determine what cloning meant for society in general. If a lamb could be cloned, could not other mammals, including humans? If so, what changes in human life would this unleash? Leon Kass (1997) wrote of the "intuitive repugnance" generated by the idea of human cloning, and he urged citizens and policymakers to respect that intuition and not allow cloning to take place. Polls taken immediately after Dolly's announced birth revealed virtually no support for cloning. In one poll, a sample of Americans was asked, "In general, do you think it is a good idea or a bad idea to clone human beings?" Fully 93 percent said it was a bad idea, 4 percent said it was a good idea, and 3 percent were not sure. Seventy-four percent believed cloning was "against God's will" and 91 percent would not clone themselves if they had the opportunity to do so (*Time* Magazine and Cable Network News 2001). Advisory bodies and professional associations surveyed in the United States revealed a nearly universal agreement that reproductive cloning would be unethical, at least at present (Eiseman 1997). In the United States three associations that included as members virtually all professionals in a position to attempt reproductive cloning—the American Society for Reproductive Medicine (ASRM), Federation of American Societies for Experimental Biology, and Biotechnology Industry Organization (BIO)—all asked their members to observe a moratorium on reproductive SCNT.

Amid widespread calls to prevent human reproductive cloning, some nations did indeed bar it, yet various constraints precluded swift and forceful action in the United States. These constraints are worthy of examination for the role they play in cloning policy in particular and in policy relating to the intersection of reproductive and genetic technologies in general. Of them, three are highlighted here. One constraint is scientific: the inclination, in a nation that values technology and its contribution to free enterprise, to regard the incremental and serendipitous nature of scientific development through trusting eyes. A second is ethical: the difficulty policymakers experience in reaching consensus about the nature of the human embryo and acting when interventions on the embryo are at issue. A third is political: the inclination in a pluralistic and free market society that prizes individual liberties toward private rather than public policy. These inclinations weave throughout policy deliberations, and they help to explain the cautious approach in the United States to moving beyond the existing regulatory model.

TECHNOLOGICAL OPTIMISM

If instant recognition of one's name is an indicator of fame, Dolly was famous beyond all hope of her lesser-known compatriots whose births were announced by scientists at the Roslin Institute at the same time as Dolly's: Cedric, Cyril, Cecil, Tuppence, Taffy, and Tweed. All of these births involved nuclear transfer, but Dolly was the only lamb of this group to have been conceived by reversing a differentiated adult somatic cell. To achieve Dolly's conception, scientists at Roslin transferred the nucleus of a differentiated body cell (in this case from mammary gland tissues of an adult ewe that had died several years earlier) to a donor egg from which the nucleus had been removed. Following an electrical charge to stimulate fusion, the egg underwent a chemical change, as it would have if a spermatozoan had entered it, and began dividing to become an embryo (Wilmut, Campbell, and Tudge 1997).

In all, scientists created 277 embryos using SCNT and transferred them to the oviducts of surrogate ewes, where the oviducts acted as "temporary incubators" to allow the embryos to develop to the more developed blastocyst stage (Wilmut, Campbell, and Tudge 2000, 185). Only twenty-nine of the original 277 embryos developed to the blastocyst stage. Scientists transferred these twenty-nine to the uteruses of thirteen surrogate ewes. One of the ewes became pregnant and gave birth to Dolly. It was, wrote Wilmut, Campbell, and Tudge (2000, 216), a "skin of the teeth success." Reproductive SCNT enabled a birth without a new combination of genes, although Dolly did inherit the cytoplasm and mitochondrial DNA of the egg donor.

In the same scientific publication introducing Dolly's birth, Wilmut and colleagues reported the births of Taffy and Tweed. The scientists cloned these lambs through the transfer of nuclei from skin fibroblast cells of sheep fetuses to enucleated eggs. This form of SCNT was less of a biological feat because the fetal somatic cells were closer to the undifferentiated state than were adult somatic cells. Scientists cloned Cecil, Cedric, Cyril, and Tuppence using nuclei transferred from a sheep embryo. Their births were less dramatic than those of Dolly, Taffy, and Tweed because these embryo cells had not yet differentiated.

While Dolly's birth may have surprised the scientific community, Dolly's developers regarded it more as a notch in an incremental series of advances. In a detailed account of the scientific history leading to Dolly's birth, Wilmut and colleagues marked as significant the births of Tracy (the first transgenic lamb) and the births of Megan and Morag (cloned from embryo cell nuclear transfer). The investigators' goal all along was to enable IGMs for commercial animal biotechnology. They aimed to flood body cells with DNA sequences that code for the desired trait (such as protein in milk) and transfer only those nuclei that took up the sequences to enucleated eggs in the nuclear transfer process. This would be considerably more efficient than traditional germ-line interventions, in which technicians inserted DNA sequences manually into the pronuclei of fertilized eggs and where, more often than not, the DNA did not integrate or express properly.

Tracy's 1990 birth illustrated the traditional approach. Here, scientists injected the gene that coded for alpha-l-antitrypsin (AAT), a protein potentially of use for treating cystic fibrosis, into the pronucleus of a fertilized egg. The resulting lamb, Tracy, successfully produced large volumes of AAT in her milk. Polly, born in 1997, illustrated the more modern approach envisioned by Wilmut and others. Researchers flooded fetal fibroblasts with a human gene and a marker gene. Using the marker DNA sequences to select the cells that took up the gene, they transferred the nuclei of these cells to enucleated eggs. From fetal cell nuclear transfer, Polly was born and she expressed the human gene (Kolata 1998a, 232). In the United States, researchers had cloned cattle from early-stage embryos in 1987 and 1989 and from later-stage embryos in 1994 (Wilmut, Campbell, and Tudge 2000, 137).

Steady incremental advances and serendipitous findings provide the raw materials for scientific discovery. Various incentives motivate those who pursue these discoveries. One is the lure of the challenge combined with personal doggedness. As Keith Campbell said of mammalian cloning, which he pursued when others asserted it could not be done, "I always believed that if you could do this in a frog, you could do it in mammals" (Specter and Kolata 1997). Other incentives are curiosity and the thrill of insight. When others proclaimed DNA a giant, dull molecule, for example, James Watson, who elucidated the structure of DNA with Francis Crick, called DNA the "most interesting molecule in all of nature" (Wilmut, Campbell, and Tudge 2000, 24).

Other incentives relate to the professional recognition that comes with pathbreaking discoveries and the association with respected and productive research teams. Economic incentives and patent opportunities are powerful motivations; Wilmut and Campbell postponed news of Dolly's birth for six months, for example, to give them time to apply for a patent for part of their cloning procedure (Specter and Kolata 1997). Other cloning investigators applied for patents for variations in the cloning method (Butler 1998). The need for novelty that underlies patent law pushes investigators to invention and discovery. Active research programs also translate to grants, improved research facilities, and other resources.

The lure of discovery extends beyond individual scientists and research facilities to a broader cultural optimism about the outcome of technological development. In the United States, habitual utilitarian calculations presume that technological growth will bring a surfeit of benefits over costs. This optimism creates the sense of an upward trajectory. With this perspective, it is anathema to limit basic or applied research, which would interfere with unforeseen benefits, acquisition of knowledge, and therapeutic applications. A sense prevails that barring nuclear transfer technology, especially if the restriction is not narrowly drawn, will produce an escalating impact. What may appear to be a simple restriction will result in significant future losses, where loss is equated with knowledge not gained. In the matter of ES cell research, for example, supporters argue that limiting SCNT technology might condemn many patients to unnecessary suffering because of lost knowledge and discoveries.

On the other hand, this perspective also suggests that research funding and other positive governmental acts will yield benefits that may not be immediately obvious. In the matter of ES cell research, supporters argued that these universal, highly pliable cells had virtually unlimited potential to address disease, promote health, and prolong life. Similar assumptions of escalating benefits fueled efforts to secure governmental funding of somatic cell gene therapy in the early 1990s. While gene therapy has not been the magic bullet some predicted, persistent researchers continue their efforts, motivated by belief in the basic premise of gene therapy.

Glenn McGee and Arthur Caplan (1999, 153) see this persistence as a "moral imperative of compassion for the sick and vulnerable." Others, such as Daniel Callahan (2000, 654), are more skeptical of what might be seen as a "research imperative." To them, technology breeds more technology. Callahan (1990, 63–65) writes of the ragged edge of medicine, in which it is expected that first one problem and then another can be resolved through medical progress. Once one problem is addressed, however, another surfaces, thus launching renewed efforts to tap down this new rough spot on the edge. The effort to smooth the edge, writes Callahan, never ends, thereby leaving a perpetually ragged edge and repeated efforts to hone the edges. While Callahan used this analogy in a critical sense, others see the effort to smooth the edge of disease as invoking the best of human nature—always fixing, always improving. Even if deleterious impacts occur, the thinking goes, new technologies can remedy the dilemmas the existing technologies wrought.

Optimism about the technological future is by no means limited to the United States, although the wealth of the country makes it an exemplar of the perspective. In the view of A. Mauron and J.-M. Thevoz (1991, 650), technological optimism is common especially in the Anglo culture, where it bespeaks a utilitarian mode of thinking in which observers "seem as a rule more confident in their ethico-legal capability to promote good and prevent evil." In countries where technological optimism undergirds the political culture, policy is more likely to promote unfettered development. Here the burden of proof for imposing barriers falls on the shoulders of those who want to limit technology. Without compelling proof to the contrary, benefits are presumed, along with the belief in the ability of the polity to manage harms. A contrary position inheres in the precautionary principle, which holds that one should not proceed if there is a risk of harm, even if that risk has not been demonstrated empirically (Nuffield Council on Bioethics 1999, 8). This presumption of harm has not prevailed as an operating principle in the United States.

PERSISTENT CONFLICT OVER EMBRYO RESEARCH

In the midst of hearings on ES cells in the U.S. Senate on April 26, 2000, a telling exchange occurred between Sens. Sam Brownback (R-KS) and Arlen Specter (R-PA). Knowing that the extraction of ES cells from donated human embryos would destroy the embryos, Sen. Brownback likened this act to "some of the things that happened in World War II" (U.S. Senate, Committee on Appropriations, Subcommittee on Labor, Health and Human Services, and Education, and Related Agencies [CA-SLHERA] 2000b, 32). He explained that the fact that the embryos were going to be destroyed anyway did not justify removing cells from the embryos in the process any more than were the Nazis justified in experimenting on people who were going to die anyway. Sen. Specter replied, "But they were living people unlike the embryos." Sen. Brownback responded, "These are living embryos. These are living embryos." A few minutes later Sen. Specter returned to the subject, saying:

> I think we do have to keep some perspective on this. I put something on this piece of paper, and I will bet no one out there can tell me what is on that piece of paper because you cannot see it. But I took my pencil and I put a dot on it. That is how big we are talking about. That is how big the human embryo is that we are talking about. In fact, in most cases you cannot even see it with the naked eye. Now . . . to equate that with the individual person that the Nazis were experimenting upon I think is to stretch the meaning of humanness and what a human being is (U.S. Senate, CA-SLHERA, 2000b, 35).

Underscoring virtually all policy discussions on SCNT are persistent, unyielding differences in the meanings individuals ascribe to human embryos. For one person, removing a cell from a human embryo is akin to removing a vital organ from a person walking down the street (U.S. Senate, CA-SLHERA 1999). For another person, the human embryo is living but is not the moral equivalent of a person who has been born (U.S. Department of Health, Education and Welfare [DHEW], Ethics Advisory Board [EAB] 1979).

Discussions about the human embryo are frequently framed in terms of the embryo's moral status. An important distinction arises between those who regard the embryo as a person with all the protections accorded fellow members of the human community and those who regard the embryo as deserving respect as a potential human being but not the same respect accorded persons. A third position, that the embryo is "just cells" and need not be accorded any extra respect, is not seriously advanced in policy discussions.

A predominant view among those who regard the embryo as sharing the moral status of children and adults is that this status begins during fertilization, when the DNA from the female and male gametes combines to create an entity with a novel genetic composition. According to Jerome Lejeune (1984, 9), when the twenty-three chromosomes from the female and the twenty-three chromosomes from the male mix, the "full genetic information, necessary and sufficient to spell out all the inborn qualities of the new individual, is gathered." He equates personhood with the formation of a unique genotype:

> Exactly as the introduction of a minicassette inside a tape recorder will allow the "re-creation" of the symphony, the information included in the 46 chromosomes (the minicassettes of the symphony of life) will be deciphered by the machinery of the cytoplasm of the fertilized egg (the tape recorder), and the new being begins to express himself as soon as he has been conceived (Lejeune 1984, 9).

For adherents of this position, the embryo is entitled to full protection from fertilization on. According to Edmund Pellegrino, the being's status does not grow as the person develops; rather, "human life is a continuum from the one cell stage to death" (NBAC 1999c, 4). From fertilization on, whatever is impermissible for a three-year-old child or a twenty-five-year-old man or a sixty-seven-year-old woman is also impermissible for a human embryo. The embryo is to be protected as an end in itself and not as a means to another end: "[A] human being from conception to death cannot be exploited for any purpose whatsoever" (McCormick 1999, 550–51, quoting Pope John Paul II). The embryo may not be willfully destroyed, even to produce a beneficial end, any more than an adult may be destroyed for another end. Embryos no longer needed or wanted by couples in fertility programs must be protected as vulnerable individuals (Doerflinger 1999, 145). An embryo cannot be destroyed "with respect." The only morally acceptable respect is that which gives the embryonic human the chance to be born. All "living member[s] of the human species," including embryos and fetuses, have a "moral claim to protection"; human life at all stages "has dignity and merits protection" (NBAC 1999c, 4).

A less frequently expressed view of those who accord the embryo the same status as persons is that the status begins later, with developmental rather than genetic individuality. The fourteenth day after fertilization is thought to be about the time an embryo, if it survives, is committed to developing into an individual. Before this time the embryo could divide to form more than one embryo or it could turn into a tumor with no developmental potential. Around the fourteenth day after fertilization, however, the microscopic embryo begins to take on signs of individuality. It has about 2,000 cells, and a primitive streak or groove starts to develop along the embryo's middle line and the "cells move from one layer to another in an organized way." The groove establishes the embryo's "head-tail and left-right orientations" and is a marking point in the embryo's development (National Institutes of Health 1994, 21, 107). According to this perspective, research can be performed on human embryos under controlled conditions until the beginning of personhood at approximately the fourteenth day after fertilization.

A sense of awe can arise in these discussions of the human embryo. To Teresa Iglesias, the embryo is "indisputably human." It is "a human being in his or her embryonic stage of existence" (Iglesias 1990, 9) that must be valued for its inherent and present self, not simply for what it can become. "In the blastocyst," writes Leon Kass, "even in the zygote, we face a mysterious and awesome power, a power governed by an immanent plan that may produce an indisputably and fully human being" (quoted in Iglesias 1990, 9).

A contrasting perspective holds that embryos have developmental potential but do not share the moral status of persons who have been born. This, too, can evoke expressions of awe. Robert Edwards, the pioneer of IVF, marveled at the human embryo outside the body and seen through the lens of a microscope. About the embryo that later became Louise Brown, Edwards said, "the last time I saw her, she was just eight cells in a test-tube. She was beautiful then, and she's still beautiful now!" (Tarin et al. 1992). Brigid Hogan, a mouse embryologist, speaks of the mystique of the mouse embryo: "It is to me the most beautiful thing in the world, quite exquisitely beautiful, and the idea that one could eventually describe how it is formed and grows just in terms of molecules and genes and pathways doesn't detract from the beauty at all, makes it more awesome, in fact" (Wade 1999, D7).

According to this view, which has variations, conception is a process, not a moment, and there is not a particular point where personhood commences. After syngamy, the fertilized egg divides into two, then four, then eight cells, and so on. Each of these early cells or blastomeres is undifferentiated (totipotent) and could, if separated, develop into individual embryos, as happens with identical twins or higher-order multiples. At this point the blastomeres are distinct totipotent cells with the zona pellucida as protective covering. After the sixteen-cell stage, the cell membranes and cytoplasm change and the cells start to adhere. They continue to divide but become smaller, and the embryo stays the same size as the cells pack together four to five days after fertilization.

As the embryo becomes a blastocyst, it has an inner cell wall and hollow center. In natural conception, the embryo implants into the uterine wall five to seven days after syngamy. Approximately two-thirds of embryos do not survive to live birth, and most are lost in the fourteen days after fertilization (American College of Obstetricians and Gynecologists, Committee on Ethics 1994). Successful implantation is the exception rather than the rule; embryo loss is normal and is even beneficial if it sloughs abnormal embryos from the body. While the early embryos have a precarious existence, this does not in itself justify the destruction of human embryos for other ends. It does, however, suggest that embryo loss is built into natural conception.

Positions about the moral status of human embryos are related but not limited to religious beliefs. The view that the embryo is a person from fertilization is associated most visibly with Roman Catholicism. For example, the Instruction for Respect on Human Life delivered from the Vatican in 1987 counsels that the embryo is to be "treated as a person from the moment of conception" (The Vatican 1987). Still, within this general viewpoint are differences among those who believe personhood starts at fertilization and those who believe it starts with the formation of the primitive streak about the fourteenth day after conception (McCormick 1999; NBAC 1999c, 8). The view that personhood begins at conception is expressed also in the Eastern Orthodox perspective, in which personhood is viewed as a process in which life is sanctified at all stages of development and in which born and unborn humans are entitled to the same respect. According to one interpretation, it is not possible to know when or how the developing human attains a soul, so it is advisable to err on the side of caution and treat the embryo with dignity and respect without interfering at any time with its development (NBAC 1999c, 33).

In contrast, under interpretations of Judaic law, the embryo outside the uterus is not different morally from eggs or spermatozoa (NBAC 1999c, 18). Embryos have potential for life but "need a little help," which is to be transferred to a woman's uterus. If the embryo implants in the uterine wall, it is a living cell and is not without protection, but its status for the first forty days is, as the fetus, "like water." This Judaic perspective accepts a growing continuum of moral status from the early stages of development to those beyond birth. Interventions can be performed on the embryo in order to advance other goals or ends, such as protecting human health. This may even include a mandate to pursue research with embryos if the studies will maintain health and life (NBAC 1999c, 17–18).

Protestant religions differ over the moral necessity of protecting embryos, and the determination is more a matter of individual conscience than denominational policy. Respect is generally accorded the embryo, but not to the same degree owed to children and adults. For example, the United Church of Christ has no official position on the embryo's status. Its General Synod passed a resolution on cloning in 1997, however, saying the embryo was to be accorded respect, although it was not the equivalent of a person (NBAC 1999c, 51). Denominations have different perspectives regarding the moral necessity of protecting embryos. Divine commands differ about the use of embryos in research along with compassion for the suffering of fellow humans and the search for life-saving therapies through research (NBAC 1999c, 48). Islamic perspectives vary between Sunni and Shi'ite schools of thought. According to some interpretations of Sunni legal thought, the developing being is ensouled when it begins moving in the fourth month of pregnancy. A Shi'ite perspective, on the other hand, holds that ensoulment inheres at the very beginning of development (NBAC 1999c, 40–42).

Differences in beliefs about the embryo, especially about whether it shares the moral status of children and adults, are basic and persistent. After reviewing diverse positions on embryo research among European states, the European Group on Ethics in Science and New Technologies (EGE) concluded that it would be more fruitful to seek accommodation among the views than consensus (European Commission, EGE 1999). Part of that accommodation is to avoid policymaking. In the United States, this means the U.S. government has historically steered clear of issues relating to interventions that lead to the destruction of human embryos, although this accommodation has been shaken by conflicts over the funding of ES cell research.

In the United States, no facet of the policy deliberations surrounding innovative reproductive technologies has been untouched by this backdrop of differing ideas and perspectives about the moral status of the human embryo. It has been said that "the politics of abortion unfolds like a Kabuki play, stylized and familiar" (Toner 2001). So too are aspects of the politics of embryo research "stylized and familiar," although ES cell issues have provoked some unusual policy positions across political parties. Still, when the time comes to translate principles to formal policy, issues relating to the status of the embryo become an inevitable part of the calculation (Annas, Caplan, and Elias 1996). The inability of policymakers to reach common ground on this matter does much to explain the difficulty in developing a cloning policy.

INCLINATION TOWARD PRIVATE POLICY

George Annas has written that "[w]e have three basic models for scientific/medical policymaking in the U.S.: the market, professional standards, and legislation. We tend to worship the first, distrust the second, and disdain the third" (U.S. Senate, CLHS-SPHS 1997a, 5). While this might overstate the case, it is certainly accurate to observe that a free marketplace is a prized goal in biotechnology research. In the area of ARTs in particular, market forces and professional standards have prevailed over legislation.

It is not surprising that an inclination toward private policy characterizes ART policy in the United States. The political system does, after all, use a complex network of mechanisms to diffuse power and to ward against centralized authority. A distrust of governmental power and support for individualism weave through policymaking, especially in matters involving families, child rearing, and reproduction. The U.S. Supreme Court has protected the right to be left alone in private matters with decisions that extend the liberty interests protected by the 5th and 14th Amendments to include end-of-life as well as beginning-of-life decision making. While a woman's liberty interest in terminating a pregnancy is not absolute, the Court has in the past two decades protected it in the face of legislative efforts to value societal interests over individual private action.

Private policy brings the expectation of minimal governmental presence in matters relating to ART practice. Alternatives to government involvement include monitoring by the profession and a distant safety net made up of tort law, licensing procedures, insurance laws, and other policies that affect the practice of medicine. The development of principles and rules of practice governing ARTs have to this point been most actively shaped by practitioners, researchers, professional associations, industry organizations, and patient advocacy groups.

Private policy is incremental and cumulative. At its most basic level, it begins in clinics, where practitioners identify clinical issues associated with new technologies. Clinic policies are written or explicit ideas about whom to accept as patients, what procedures to offer, and what to present in the informed consent process. These policies involve discretionary judgments about when and how to initiate new technologies. In another stage of private policy, clinic policies are shared across clinics. Here a diffusion of innovation can take place when pioneering clinics provide procedural models to which other clinics may look in developing their own policies. When such modeling takes place, areas of consensus emerge and are expressed in written documents such as ethics committee statements of fertility societies. The more that rules are specified, shared, and based on recognized criteria, the closer they come to being part of a private policy (Bonnicksen 2001b, 25).

For ARTs, where the government has traditionally not been active, professional associations have produced guidance documents, position statements by ethics committees, and relatively formal policies. For example, in response to inadequate ART data collection, the American Fertility Society (now the ASRM) formed a group, the Society for Assisted Reproductive Technologies (SART), to encourage fertility clinics to report success rates and other data (Garcia 1998, 624). The SART published its first report in the association's journal, *Fertility and Sterility*, summarizing data on practices and outcomes in 1985 and 1986 from forty-one fertility clinics (Steinberg et al. 1998, 619). Ten years later, the annual report covered data on over 65,000 ART cycles initiated in 300 clinics in the United States in 1996 (SART and ASRM 1999). Nearly all IVF clinics in the United States are SART members, and membership brings with it the obligation to submit data to the ASRM/SART registry, apply for laboratory accreditation, and accept site visits to monitor data gathering (Steinberg et al. 1998, 619).

The private policy model causes concern about whether the "medical profession, no matter how well meaning, has the ability to monitor itself" (C. Cohen 1997, 352). As sellers of a service or product, clinicians are not unbiased arbiters, nor is it clear how much they are guided by recommendations of professional associations. Various commentators have recommended new legislation to protect children, gamete and embryo donors, and families (C. Cohen 1997, 362). For example, the ISLAT Working Group, located at the Institute for Science, Law, and Technology (ISLAT) at the Illinois Institute of Technology (ISLAT Working Group 1998), and George Annas (1998a, 938), a law professor, call for national standards governing such things as record keeping and informed consent procedures.

Still, professional associations have played an influential role in ART policymaking. Although without legal enforcement power, they assert authority through appeals to ethical behavior and membership sanctions. Moreover, industry and government have worked together in informal policy development. For example, over time, representatives from the private sector worked with Sen. Ron Wyden (D-OR) and other members of Congress to craft the *Fertility Clinic Success Rate and Certification Act of 1992* (FCSRCA), which arose out of the SART data-gathering initiative. This single federal law related to ART practice directed the Centers for Disease Control and Prevention (CDC) to develop model standards to accredit fertility laboratories, where eggs, spermatozoa, and embryos are handled. The CDC released its model certification program in 1999, and the program is consistent with standards developed earlier in the private sector (ASRM 1999). The law's purpose was minimal. It was intended to give states a model of reporting practices to consider adopting, not to mandate standards (C. Cohen 1997, 351). The FCSRCA makes the CDC the first federal agency to set standards for embryo laboratories (ASRM 1999), which is significant because not all of the approximately 350 embryo laboratories in the United States are accredited or certified (Smith 2000, 174). Although the program was not funded at first, Congress later allocated $1 million to it (C. Cohen 1997, 351).

Informal policymaking takes other forms as well. For example, the SART founded the National Coalition for Oversight of the Assisted Reproductive Technologies, which invites members from SART, ASRM, RESOLVE (an infertility support group), the CDC, FDA, and Federal Trade Commission to meet regularly to identify issues and discuss self-regulation (McNamee 2000). In addition, the ASRM, BIO, and other organizations have sent representatives to testify in congressional hearings on cloning with proposals for modifying bills to focus prohibitions on as narrow a zone of research as possible.

While national ART legislation may yet be initiated, little in the historic tradition indicates that this is likely. It is noteworthy that the United States is not alone in its inclination toward private policy. When Howard Jones, Jr., and Jean Cohen (1991) coordinated a survey of ART practitioners in thirty-eight nations, over half responded they had no national ART legislation. While twenty nations did have a national statute setting forth a framework, eleven, including the United States, relied on voluntary adherence to guidelines, and seven had neither statute nor guidelines. This finding did not change appreciably in a repeat survey in 2000 (Jones and Cohen 2001).

CONCLUSIONS

Public policy has been compared to a primeval soup in which ideas, bills, speeches, proposals, and amendments are floated, drafted, and floated again (Kingdon 1984, 123). If this is the case, policy for reproductive SCNT is particularly like a French soup, the pot-au-feu, which cooks on the fire indefinitely. Family members add ingredients to the pot daily and remove cups for their meals but the pot is never totally emptied and the base simmers for years. Cloning is like a new ingredient added to a base of long-simmering values. Optimism about the technological future, an inclination not to impose public controls on research and development, and unresolved issues about the beginnings of life all work against quick, straightforward congressional action.

Of the many approaches to a cloning policy, four are categorized here. One is legislation with a narrow arc. Supporters of this approach would regard the risks of reproductive cloning as so significant that steps must be taken to ensure cloning does not take place. The usual mechanisms are not sufficient, under this perspective; a new law, with penalties attached that bar human reproductive SCNT, is considered the most efficient and effective way of discouraging the act. With the attention focused on reproductive SCNT only, the law would target only a narrow act—the transfer of an embryo created through SCNT to a woman's uterus for possible pregnancy.

A second approach is legislation with a broad arc. Supporters of this approach would be so wary of reproductive SCNT that they aim to ban any creation of an embryo through SCNT, even if that embryo is never transferred to a woman's uterus. From this perspective, practice in creating embryos through SCNT will pose what might become an irresistible temptation one day to use the technique for reproduction. Under this approach, all human SCNT is forbidden, even for research purposes. Another aim of supporters of this approach may be to limit the use of embryos in research in general.

A third approach is to rely on the current regulatory model. Supporters would posit that existing features of the policy apparatus—including moral persuasion, guidelines from professional associations, and a government safety net made up of tort actions, licensing laws, the FCSRCA, and FDA oversight—are sufficient for monitoring reproductive SCNT. This approach may also reveal less worry about the harms of reproductive SCNT (Robertson 1998, 1439).

A fourth approach also relies on existing mechanisms but with adjustments and refinements. Supporters would regard some public adjustments as appropriate, such as solidifying FDA jurisdiction over reproductive SCNT, extending federal funding and oversight, and providing a forum for deliberations about innovative ARTs. The adjustments may or may not require legislative action.

This chapter reviewed features of the policy context that help explain why changes to the status quo are elusive and why innovative reproductive technologies have traditionally been insulated from governmental restrictions. Chapters 3, 4, and 5 review congressional efforts to enact legislation between 1997 and 2000. These efforts reveal a cautious orientation to a contentious technology. Partly for the reasons reviewed in this chapter, this orientation reflects political reality.

CHAPTER 3

ATTEMPTS TO LEGISLATE: U.S. CONGRESS, 1997

With widespread concerns in 1997 about reproductive SCNT, it made sense to turn to the U.S. Congress as a forum for deliberation. The national legislature provides a central place and structure for open debate and its staff members have access to the research services needed for a serious exploration of scientific issues. For something that strikes the sense of human identity as intimately as reproductive SCNT, resort to deliberations in a public institution that are taped on C-SPAN, recorded in minute detail in the *Congressional Record*, and available for timely access on the Internet has distinct merit. In addition, the issue itself is political, and in the legislative arena the political dimensions can be recognized and confronted.

On the other hand, legislative politics can skew a discussion into a struggle over competing interests with remarkable speed. When that discussion involves human embryos, politics take on a special intensity. The appearance of both reproductive SCNT and embryo research issues produced conflict on Capitol Hill in 1997. At the same time, during this year Congress and the NBAC deliberately sifted through issues and gave voice to basic policy options.

EARLY ACTIONS AND INFORMATION GATHERING

In 1997 the Clinton administration took immediate steps to find out more about what had happened and to distance the government from human reproductive cloning. First, three days after Dolly's announced birth, President Clinton set fact finding into motion by asking the NBAC to conduct a "thorough review" of cloning's legal and ethical issues (Clinton 1997a). In 1995, Clinton had established the NBAC in the Office of Science and Technology Policy as a national forum for exploring ethical issues in medicine, particularly those raised by medical research (President, Executive Order 1995). The NBAC had only started meeting in October 1996 and lacked an executive director when given its cloning charge. Eighteen experts and consumer representatives appointed by the president sat on the commission, with Harold Shapiro, president of Yale University, as the chair. Originally a "little-known" panel set up to review issues relating to medical research and genetic information with the expectation it would expire in October 1997, the NBAC was suddenly thrust into a highly public role (Kolata 1997a, B9). Clinton gave the commission ninety days to complete its review, a deadline later extended by two weeks.

Second, within a week, Clinton disallowed any financial support of human cloning by directing the heads of federal agencies not to allocate federal funds "for cloning of human beings or from supporting efforts by their own scientists to clone humans" (NBAC 1997a). This was largely a symbolic act because the federal government already barred funding of embryo research and because it was unlikely scientists would attempt to clone a human being, much less succeed at it. Still, the statement sent a message of misgivings about cloning, made explicit the funding ban, and conveyed that the government was taking steps in light of public concern.

Third, Clinton urged privately funded researchers, who would not be sanctioned by a funding withdrawal, to impose and respect a voluntary moratorium on the cloning of human beings and to abide by the same restrictions as federally funded researchers. Joined at a pres-

idential press conference by Department of Health and Human Ser-
vices (DHHS) Secretary Donna Shalala, National Institutes of
Health (NIH) Director Harold Varmus, NBAC Chair Harold
Shapiro, and the President's Advisor on Science and Technology Jack
Gibbons, Clinton said:

> I am urging the entire scientific and medical community, every foun-
> dation, every university, every industry that supports work in this area
> to heed the federal government's example. I'm asking for a voluntary
> moratorium on the cloning of human beings until our Bioethics Advi-
> sory Commission and our entire nation have had a real chance to un-
> derstand and debate the profound ethical implications of the latest ad-
> vances (Clinton, 1997b).

On Capitol Hill, members of Congress introduced three bills to
prevent human cloning. On the day the report of Dolly's birth was
published in *Nature*, Sen. Christopher (Kit) Bond (R-MO), a former governor of Missouri, introduced S. 368 (U.S. Senate 1997).
The bill would make permanent the ban on federal funds for
cloning an individual. The bill defined cloning as the replication of
an individual by removing "a cell with genetic material and cultivating that cell through stages into a new human individual." Bond intended to "send a clear signal" that human cloning, a "morally reprehensible technology," would not be tolerated (*Cong. Rec.* 1997,
S1734).

The language of S. 368 echoed Clinton's directive, except it would
impose a permanent rather than temporary ban on federal funds. But
Bond's remarks on the Senate floor indicated he wanted to bar the
funding of human cloning and human cloning research, which went
beyond Clinton's call for a moratorium on funding the "cloning of
human beings." Bond argued there was precedent for S. 368. Clinton
had barred federal funding of human cloning, and the Human Embryo Research Panel (HERP) had recommended in its 1994 report
that cloning would not be an ethically acceptable intervention on
human embryos (NIH 1994). Bond said it was self-evident that
cloning was unacceptable and the NBAC charge was superfluous: "I
do not think we need to study this. There are some aspects of life
which simply ought to be off limits to science." Plant or animal
cloning was not a problem, Bond argued, but creating another

human being through cloning is where "we must draw the line" (*Cong. Rec.* 1997, S1734).

Rep. Vernon Ehlers (R-MI), a former college professor who received a Ph.D. in nuclear physics in 1960, introduced two bills on March 5, 1997. The first, H.R. 922, would, like S. 368, forbid federal funds for cloning a human being (U.S. House 1997b):

> None of the funds made available in any Federal law may be expended to conduct or support any project of research that involves the use of a human somatic cell for the process of producing a human clone.

The second bill, H.R. 923, the *Human Cloning Prohibition Act of 1997*, would make cloning a human being through reproductive SCNT illegal and impose a $5,000 civil penalty for violating the law (U.S. House 1997c). As defined, the bill would make it "unlawful for any person to use a human somatic cell for the process of producing a human clone."

Ehlers wanted to ban human cloning to prevent a backlash that might endanger acceptable animal cloning research (Seelye 1997, A10). He also had reservations about the safety of human cloning ("the failed experiments, the clones that go wrong"), the "profound issues of ethics, morality, theology, and religious belief," and the distance cloning would inject between marriage and ordinary methods of conception (*Cong. Rec.* 1997, H713–14). Ehlers' bills presented two methods of drawing lines: one to deny funds for human cloning research and the other to outlaw the act of cloning a human being. The bills on the table varied by the targeted act, method of enforcement, and duration (see Table 3.1).

TABLE 3.1 Proposed Legislation in U.S. Congress, March 1997

Proposal	Targeted Act	Method	Duration
S. 368	Research on cloning a human being	No federal funding	Permanent
H.R. 922	Research using a somatic cell to produce a human clone	No federal funding	Permanent
H.R. 923	Using a somatic cell to produce a human clone	Civil penalty of $5,000	Permanent

CONGRESSIONAL HEARINGS

On March 5, 1997, the House Committee on Science held the first of five congressional hearings designed to explore issues relating to reproductive cloning. The committee's Subcommittee on Technology convened a hearing (U.S. Committee on Science, Subcommittee on Technology [CS-ST] 1997a) to consider H.R. 922's provision permanently to ban federal funding for human cloning (U.S. House 1997a). A standing room only crowd lined the committee room when subcommittee chair Constance Morella (D-MD) convened the hearing. The hearing featured five witnesses representing science, bioethics, and the biotechnology industry. Morella and her colleagues set the tone by distinguishing between the cloning of humans, which they rejected, and ongoing research in animal biotechnology, which they supported.

Morella, whose district included Montgomery County, home of the NIH and a large concentration of biotechnology firms, cautioned that it was important to protect "potentially positive scientific developments" amid efforts to proscribe human cloning. She argued that animal cloning held promise for medical research, including the development of new drugs and animal organs for transplantation, and she urged lawmakers not to restrict promising science when proscribing human cloning. She noted that the government had taken steps to discourage cloning, including a charge to the NBAC, a presidential directive that no federal agencies should fund research leading to human cloning, and the voluntary moratorium on privately funded researchers urged by the president.

Subcommittee member George E. Brown, Jr. (D-CA) reminded his colleagues that cloning research with animals had been ongoing for some time and that practical uses of cloning with animals held promise. The discussions should go beyond cloning, he thought, and initiate a national dialogue on research and public policy. F. James Sensenbrenner, Jr. (R-WI) added it was important to allow biotechnology research to proceed at the same time steps were taken to make sure humans were not cloned. "We should not," he stated, "let our concerns over the potential of cloning human beings override the fact that we've got to continue biological research in these areas [of biotechnology] so that we can be healthier, and live longer lives, have better food, and have a higher quality of life."

The hearing was designed to inform committee members of cloning in animals and to review the policy implications of cloning. Witnesses were both wary about human cloning and supportive of legitimate research in biotechnology. Harold E. Varmus, director of the NIH, reviewed the science of animal cloning and described the promise it held for the agriculture industry, particularly when cloning and transgenic research were combined. Nuclear transfer, in which human cells are reprogrammed but no embryos are transferred for pregnancy, held hope for new ways to treat disease. On the prospect of reproductive SCNT to create humans, he wondered if it might be permissible in infrequent situations, subject to careful regulation. He welcomed the airing of issues in Congress and in the NBAC.

A geneticist with the U.S. Department of Agriculture said researchers at the department had not been involved with SCNT research with animals. He acknowledged the accomplishments of the researchers in Scotland and talked about the promise of transgenic research with animals. A scientist with the Oregon Regional Primate Research Center shared news of her research cloning Rhesus monkeys by transferring nuclei from embryonic cells, and she told of the promise of the cloning research. An executive at Genzyme Transgenics described how cloning could facilitate transgenic research by producing many offspring from a female transgenic animal. He urged committee members not to rush to judgment in a way that would produce bad policy. Research with therapeutic benefits should be protected.

Thomas Murray, a bioethicist who was also an NBAC member, urged an understanding of the facts of animal and human cloning, with the supposition that "good ethics begin with good facts." He said it was important to understand the reasons for the current moral objections to and values challenged by cloning. Existing laws that could relate to cloning should be examined to see whether they could be extended to give the desired protection. He urged committee members not to take irreversible action before the NBAC completed its deliberations and issued recommendations. He called for a realistic assessment of what cloning can and cannot do, specifically explaining the replication of an existing human being as one thing cloning cannot do. A clone of Mel Gibson would look like Mel Gibson, he said, but the clone would be very different from the Mel Gibson loved by his fans.

The Senate convened its first hearing on cloning a week later, on March 12, 1997, in the Subcommittee on Public Health and Safety of the Committee on Labor and Human Resources (U.S. Senate 1997a). Subcommittee chair William Frist (R-TN) noted that this was the first time in the two and a half weeks since Dolly's announced birth that a representative from NBAC, a scientist involved in the Dolly experiment that produced Dolly, and members of the biotechnology community had sat in a single forum. He hoped this would set the stage for "an open, a reasoned, and a balanced discussion of the issue of cloning." A former heart surgeon, Frist remembered fears about heart transplantation in the 1960s and the importance of balanced and public discussions in promoting public understanding. The hearing was devoted to fact-finding and to explicating the issues raised by cloning.

Before three panels of experts addressed the subcommittee, various senators spoke. Sens. Ted Kennedy (D-MA) and Christopher Bond foreshadowed differences that would reappear a year later. Noting that the "scientist who cloned Dolly has broken the biological equivalent of the sound barrier," Kennedy endorsed a cloning moratorium pending the NBAC review. Bond aimed at permanence and endorsed the long-term ban S. 368 would place on the use of federal money for human cloning.

On the first panel, Harold Varmus talked about the science of cloning. He and Ian Wilmut, the embryologist with the Roslin Institute in Scotland who generated Dolly, spoke about applications of cloning technology for animals. He cautioned that legislation is "of course, very difficult to reverse," and he advised care inasmuch as we are "not in a moment of crisis." Three law professors specializing in bioethics made up the second panel. One, a member of NBAC, gave an update on the issues being considered by the commissioners. A second argued that cloning would "cross a boundary that represents a difference in kind, rather than degree, in human reproduction" and that there were no good reasons to clone a human being. He urged Congress to use cloning as an opportunity to "establish a new regulatory framework for novel and extreme human experiments." A third speaker encouraged collaboration among federal agencies such as the FDA, NIH, CDC, and Department of Agriculture in response to cloning. The third panel featured representatives from industry who spoke about biotechnology's promise for medicine, especially when combined with transgenic technologies.

NATIONAL BIOETHICS ADVISORY COMMISSION: MEETINGS AND REPORT

After the initial round of bills and hearings, activity declined in Congress as members awaited the results of the NBAC's deliberations. The NBAC had until June to produce a report. The commissioners accelerated their schedule in order to have a report ready in time, meeting March 13–14, April 13, May 2, and May 17. They called fifteen witnesses (twelve in the first meeting) and commissioned eight background papers on animal cloning research, embryo research, the views of professional societies, religious perspectives, ethical issues, legal status, international perspectives, and research moratoria.

Despite the NBAC's tight time frame, its meetings were more leisurely than congressional hearings, where speakers observed five-minute limits for their oral presentations. The NBAC's more reflective testimony and active question-and-answer sessions advanced the NBAC's mission not only to reach conclusions but also to write a report. Shapiro likened this to writing a novel where the commissioners did not know what the story line or conclusion would be. While members of Congress could introduce a skeletal bill and know that details would be worked out later, the NBAC had to produce a written text with background material, recommendations, and justifications for the recommendations. The members' task was to produce an even-handed exposition based on their own understanding, anticipate and address arguments and counterarguments, and reach conclusions. As one speaker said, the NBAC needed to "hear the various voices" in society but at some point it also had "to take a step."

The NBAC's first meeting on March 13–14 started with a plan for proceeding: four categories or "buckets" of knowledge (philosophy, biology, law, and policy) would be created with individual commissioners at the helm of each (NBAC 1997b). The subgroups would discuss issues in depth and write draft sections of the final report, although the buckets would overlap and information and ideas would be moved from one to another. Next, members who had testified or been present at the first congressional hearings reported on their observations, revealing a cross-fertilization between Congress and the NBAC. They reported that scientists who testified in Congress did not foresee human cloning in the near future.

In the following hours, NBAC members listened to and queried twelve experts who had been selected to give presentations on the basis of their experience in biomedical ethics and the varied perspectives they were expected to represent. One NBAC member later reflected that the range, thoughtfulness, and quality of presentations were an "extraordinarily effective way to begin a kind of national conversation about the ethics of human cloning" (U.S. House, CS-ST 1997b). On the first day, NBAC members heard from a geneticist who apprised them about the science of cloning, told why the process was inefficient, and identified cloning's risks. A theology professor gave a perspective from Roman Catholicism in which she urged viewing cloning in a "broad and humanistic context" in which "questions of the common good" were weighed.

A Roman Catholic priest next spoke of cloning from the perspective of the Vatican's 1987 Instruction. Cloning was "entirely unsuitable," he said, because it violated human dignity by "exceeding the limits of the delegated dominion given to the human race." In addition, it was separate from sexual intercourse, a problem of all assisted reproductive technologies. It was more problematic than existing ARTs because "it represents a greater attempt to control the output . . . by already specifying the genome." He urged the commissioners to find out what values were common and to give them priorities. A Protestant theologian then spoke of the need to evaluate cloning by looking to what is good for the child, who is a "gift" from God.

On the second day, two professors of religion spoke of Judaic law and a third discussed Islamic interpretations of cloning. Neither of the Jewish witnesses condemned cloning; in fact, both saw merit in it. One spoke of the partnership with God in creation and of the Jewish tradition of aggressively "trying to improve a person's medical situation." Trying to change infertility or other medical situations is permissible as long as people do not shift from acting as God's agent to playing God themselves. The speaker thought it better to allow cloning with restrictions than to leave it to the discretion of those who have vested interests in it. The second speaker interpreted Jewish perspectives referring to God's "commandment" to master the earth. He thought cloning could be justified by the sanctity of life, in which people have a need for immortality though descendants. He thought cloning might be justifiable if, for example, only one person in a family survived the Holocaust and wanted to retain the family's genetic line.

A scholar of Islam noted the unusual situation in which scholars of Islam, Judaism, and Christianity were all at the same forum discussing views on human reproduction. He hoped this would launch a partnership in the search for "meaningful ways to prevent abuse of modern biomedical technology." He cautioned that human cloning had not been discussed, as far as he knew, in Islamic thought, but that it would encompass differing views, not the least because of differences between the Sunni and Shi'ite Islamic traditions. Interpretations of the Koran suggest that human beings can intervene in works of nature, including procreation. Of embryo twinning to help an infertile married couple conceive (he focused on twinning rather SCNT), he said this would be permissible if kept within marriage and if the child's lineage were kept intact according to religious precepts.

The next four witnesses spoke of cloning's risks and benefits. John Robertson, a law professor, expressed concern that the alleged harms of cloning revolved around moral questions and were symbolic rather than tangible. He did not see concrete harms to the child, family, or society. Moreover, he argued, "good uses can be imagined." Reproductive cloning was not necessarily different from other assisted reproductive technologies and might, in fact, be less radical than germline genetic interventions because it would replicate but not alter a genome. The starting presumption should be that married couples have a freedom to conceive. When harms and benefits are weighed against this backdrop of reproductive liberty, it is not clear that cloning should be restricted. Symbolic harms are not enough to warrant limiting a reproductive technology, especially when that technology might bring benefits.

Ruth Macklin, a bioethics professor, also challenged the alleged harm of cloning. She was not persuaded that replicating a genome to produce a child violated anyone's rights. The child would not necessarily be harmed and any psychological burdens of knowing that the child had been cloned did not seem to be of "such magnitude that they would outweigh the benefit of life itself." An oft-stated risk of cloning was that parents might try to use the cells from a dying child to generate another child with the same genome. It was not clear to

Macklin that this would be any more harmful than parents conceiving a child the usual way as solace when they lost a child. The outcome of the event in either case would depend on the family's child-rearing practices. To outlaw cloning, one would need "to specify the precise nature of the wrong done either to the individual from whom a clone is derived or to the resulting cloned person."

When cloning is said to violate human dignity, Macklin asserted, one must ask for a "precise account" of this violation. Dignity is a "fuzzy concept," and it can easily "substitute for empirical evidence that is lacking or sound arguments that cannot be mustered." If cloning's objectors "can identify no greater harm than a supposed affront to the dignity of the human species, that is a flimsy basis on which to erect barriers to scientific research and its applications."

Leon Kass, a physician and bioethicist, presented a contrasting perspective. Where Robertson and Macklin had started with a presumption favoring reproductive liberty, Kass started with a presumption that cloning was fundamentally wrong. Cloning is not a variation on assisted reproductive technologies, he asserted. It is "radically new" and the "stakes here are very high." Cloning has provoked a searing revulsion that is a barometer about what is right and what is wrong. "Repugnance is often the emotional bearer of deep wisdom." Cloning repels us not because it is strange or novel but because "we intuit and feel immediately and without argument the violation of things we rightfully hold dear."

To Kass, there is no compelling reason to use cloning to bring humans into the world. Moreover, it would be an "unethical experiment on the child to be" who could not consent to be conceived in this way. Second, it would create "serious issues of identity and individuality that would impose psychological burdens on the child." Third, it would turn procreation into manufacturing. Even if the children were deeply loved, they still would be artifacts, with the "profoundly dehumanizing" impact of that arrangement. Fourth, it would "aggravate a profound mischief" about the reasons for having children in which "overbearing parents" select the child's genotype and expect "that this blueprint of a past life ought to be controlling of a life that is to come." Such expectations make cloning "inherently despotic." With harms so clear and profound, the only recourse for cloning is to initiate a "unilateral national ban at a minimum."

James Nelson, a professor of bioethics, spoke of "worrisome scenarios" about cloning's impact on the family and about the importance it places on biological relatedness. He thought cloning warranted "prudent judgment." That judgment suggested that other goals and research should have priority over cloning. Five members of the audience gave brief presentations at the meeting.

By the next meeting, on April 13, the commissioners had engaged in considerable discussion among themselves (NBAC 1997c). Following presentations by two scientists, the NBAC members took part in an active interchange as leaders of the ethics, science, and policy "buckets" reported on discussions and draft conclusions reached in their subgroups. The NBAC was grappling with four separate concepts: reproductive rights, benefits, harms, and social values. Among other things, the commissioners discussed what form their opening position should take. With reproduction involved, it would make sense to begin with the idea of liberty and then look to the harms and benefits. Yet should one start with a presumption of liberty and place the burden on those who would limit it by restricting cloning? Or should one start with a presumption of injury and place the burden on those who want to engage in cloning to show a compelling reason for doing so? Where should the default lie?

The commissioners had begun narrowing their focus to the "baby making" rather than research aspect of cloning. The matter of research on embryos had been thoroughly studied three years before in the 1994 HERP report, the commissioners noted, and they did not see the need in the short time allotted for the cloning report to reintroduce the issues raised by embryo research. The members had also started to identify policy options. They asked what level of ethical concern was enough to justify restrictive options. They returned to the matter of cloning's particular harms. Among those frequently heard were the genetic control of cloning, confusing impact on relations within families, and narcissism that would motivate cloning. They sought answers to the immediate negative reaction to cloning. "Why did it make such a fuss? Why did it strike such a chord?"

The leaders of the law and policy group identified several options, from least to most restrictive: (1) allow cloning research and federal funding, (2) allow cloning research but disallow federal funding, (3) allow cloning with restrictions, giving it conditional permissibility, and (4) prohibit cloning by state or federal law. They suggested that funding cloning might actually put a brake on the research because funding would bring stringent regulations with it. Commissioners thought that a federal body such as the Recombinant DNA Advisory Committee (RAC) or the FDA might play an oversight role.

At the May 2 meeting, NBAC members focused on policy options (NBAC 1997d). They heard from Elisa Eiseman, who described the results of a survey of professional societies and associations about the science of human SCNT and the ethical and policy issues associated with it. Representatives from thirty-two associations had responded to the questionnaire and expressed views about the need to protect basic biological research on development. While they felt that practitioners should not attempt reproductive cloning at present, they supported voluntary measures rather than restrictive legislation.

At this meeting, the NBAC reinforced its decision to focus on the unique ethical issues raised by reproductive SCNT rather than on existing issues related to embryo research. Shapiro did not think this was the right time to "re-engage" embryo research issues and no pressing reason existed to do so. After the HERP issued its report three years earlier, the president and Congress, contrary to HERP recommendations, had disallowed federal funds for studies in which embryos were generated for research purposes.

After NBAC members decided they would concentrate on cloning, they began to construct a bottom line. The presidential moratorium on funding the cloning of a human and the voluntary moratorium urged for researchers in the private sector should continue, they thought. To enforce the private sector moratorium, it might be possible to suspend the licenses of physicians who disregarded the moratorium or rely on peer pressure and exhortations among physicians. Legislation would have the advantage of sending a strong and clear anticloning message, but it would be hard to reverse. Any legislation would need a sunset clause, members agreed, to allow flexibility if judgments about safety and ethics changed. The commissioners wondered about international reactions if the United States took no action on cloning. By the end of the meeting, the group was increasingly open to some form of legislation with a sunset clause.

In May, Shapiro requested and received a short continuation in order to fulfill the commission's "unusually challenging assignment" (Shapiro 1997, 195). On June 7, the NBAC convened for a final meeting to work details of the final report. Then, on June 9, with most NBAC members present, Shapiro gave the commission's report to President Clinton, Vice President Albert Gore, DHHS Secretary Donna Shalala, and NIH Director Harold Varmus in a ceremony at the White House Rose Garden (Clinton and Gore 1997). Clinton commended the NBAC on its "truly careful, insightful, and remarkable job" in producing its report on "an extremely complex issue at an extremely fast pace." He spoke of the benefits of science and technology as well as the need for protection from their harms. He distinguished between cloning cells and genes, which do not raise serious ethical issues, and cloning human beings, which do.

Gone from the 110-page report was talk of knowledge buckets and baby making (NBAC 1997). This succinct report included chapters on the scientific, religious, ethical, and legal and policy considerations of cloning. The commissioners did not revisit the embryo research issue, having focused on the impact of cloning on families and individuals. Creating embryos through SCNT for research raised no issues beyond those raised by the generation of embryos for other forms of research. Transferring embryos generated through SCNT to a woman's uterus to create a cloned person would, however. A delicate balancing was at stake. Cloning raised concerns about eugenics and treating people as objects, yet procreative liberty warranted protection as did the future of biomedical advance.

Against these suppositions, the NBAC drew five conclusions. First, it was morally unacceptable to use SCNT to generate babies because doing so would pose unacceptable safety risks for the fetus and child. As a consequence, the moratorium on federal funding to create a child through reproductive SCNT should continue, and all researchers, privately as well as publicly funded, should refrain from attempting reproductive SCNT. Professional societies should make it clear that using reproductive SCNT to conceive children would be an "irresponsible, unethical, and unprofessional act."

Second, the government should enact a law to forbid any attempt to create a child through reproductive SCNT. A national law would have several advantages, according to the NBAC. It would (1) include all researchers and persons in clinics performing procedures that are not part of research, (2) be more efficient than relying on professional societies and medical associations, (3) be preferable to ambiguous state laws, (4) discourage researchers "shopping" from state to state to find permissible laws, and (5) act as an effective deterrent because of the penalties imposed. This law (and any laws passed by the states) should have a sunset period of three to five years. An oversight body should be responsible for evaluating and reporting on cloning before the sunset period ends in order to guide policy at that point.

Third, any law should be carefully written so that restrictions do not interfere with other scientific research. No new policies are needed for human DNA cloning or animal cloning. If no law is enacted, then any clinical use of cloning must follow existing procedures protecting human research subjects. The United States should cooperate with other national and international bodies in enforcing their policies.

Fourth, given the deep moral divisions about reproductive cloning, the government should encourage deliberation in the event safety concerns one day are met. It is timely to accumulate data about cloning and to engage in a fuller debate. Participants in this debate should aim for "moral agreement," and if this is not achievable, the aim should be for "mutual respect" (Shapiro 1997, 196). Fifth, federal departments and agencies should cooperate to inform the public about genetics and other biomedical developments.

The NBAC's recommendations were both more and less restrictive than H.R. 922 and S. 368. They were more restrictive because they would forbid reproductive cloning in addition to withholding funding. They also would apply to researchers in the private as well as public sectors. The recommendations were less restrictive than congressional bills because they advocated a temporary moratorium on funding rather than a permanent ban, and they introduced a sunset clause. They targeted reproductive SCNT and left research involving SCNT alone. They carefully defined reproductive SCNT in order to narrow the range of affected research, and they added a protection clause for other scientific research.

PROPOSED LEGISLATION FROM THE PRESIDENT

The day after he accepted the NBAC's report, President Clinton sent to Congress a bill, the *Cloning Prohibition Act of 1997* (U.S. House 1997a). The most detailed proposal to that point, it complemented NBAC's recommendations. The administration's bill would bar anyone in the country, privately or publicly funded, from attempting to

TABLE 3.2 Proposed Legislation in U.S. Congress, August 1997

Proposal	Targeted Act	Method	Duration	Research Protection	Oversight
S. 368	Research on cloning a human being	No federal funding	Permanent	—	—
H.R. 922	Research using a somatic cell to produce a human clone	No federal funding	Permanent	—	—
H.R. 923	Using a somatic cell to produce a human clone	Civil penalty of $5,000	Permanent	—	—
Clinton proposal, H. Doc. 105-97	Using SCNT to produce a human clone	Civil penalty of $250,000	3 to 5 years	Yes	NBAC

create a baby through SCNT. It targeted the act of embryo transfer to a woman's uterus rather than SCNT research (see Table 3.2). It included a clause explictly protecting SCNT research on animals, added a five-year sunset clause, authorized the NBAC to continue for five years, and stipulated that the NBAC would continue to review cloning's scientific and ethical issues. It proposed a $250,000 penalty for violating the law and gave the Attorney General the sole authority to initiate a civil action to prevent a threatened violation.

ADDITIONAL HEARINGS

Three days after the NBAC issued its report, Congress held a hearing to review the NBAC's recommendations (U.S. House, CS-ST 1997b). The House Subcommittee on Technology of the Committee on Science held the first hearing after the NBAC report, just as it had been the first to hold a hearing after Dolly's announced birth. As earlier, the exchange was congenial, with members seeking information about the NBAC report as it considered H.R. 922.

Subcommittee chair Morella praised the NBAC for issuing its report under a tight time frame. She, but not all committee members, endorsed the NBAC's conclusion that research into human SCNT was ethically acceptable as long as no cloned embryos were transferred to a woman's uterus. Harold Varmus, Shapiro, and two NBAC members testified. Shapiro defended the NBAC's decision to focus on ethical issues that would be raised by the transfer of the embryo to a woman's uterus and not to examine embryo research. First, issues associated with embryo research had been recently covered by the HERP, which was formed by the NIH in the early 1990s to consider the matter of funding embryo research. Second, the president did not ask NBAC to consider embryo research, so doing so would exceed its purview. Third, embryo research policies were already in place: the president and Congress had directed no federal funds to be used for studies in which embryos were created for research. Thus, NBAC dealt only with cloning to create human beings. On this matter it recommended that Congress enact legislation to make cloning illegal.

During the course of the hearing, Ehlers, the sponsor of H.R. 922, said he agreed that legitimate research should proceed, but he anticipated disagreement ahead. As Ehlers queried NBAC members, it became clear that a major disagreement would revolve around embryo research. The NBAC believed the creation of embryos through SCNT and the transfer of them to make a baby were separate matters subject to separate policies. Ehlers and other members of the committee thought the matters could not be separated for policy purposes. Another area of disagreement was whether limits on reproductive SCNT should be temporary (NBAC) or permanent (Ehlers).

The Senate Subcommittee on Public Health and Safety of the Committee on Labor and Human Resources held a hearing to explore the ethical and religious aspects of cloning on June 17, 1997 (U.S. Senate, CLHS-SPHS 1997b). Sen. Frist convened the hearing by expressing his moral concerns about the adequacy of temporary moves taken so far. Clinton's directives left open the possibility of reproductive SCNT in the private sector, policed only by a call for a voluntary moratorium. The NBAC was silent on embryo creation, although it called for a ban on transferring embryos generated this way. The March 12 hearing had been about science. This hearing was designed to explore the morality of cloning, including religious perspectives.

The first panel of experts addressed religion and cloning. James Childress, a professor of religious studies and a member of the

NBAC, defended the NBAC's conclusion that cloning was unethical at present because of its unsettled safety. He asserted that safety was indeed a moral as well as a scientific consideration based on the "fundamental ethical obligation not to harm children." Childress also defended the NBAC's use of religious perspectives, which had been criticized by some who thought religion should not be a part of public policymaking and who wondered why an entire chapter was devoted to religion in the final report. According to Childress, religious perspectives were important because they affect the moral positions taken by individuals. Moreover, religious traditions affect values and generate moral discourse. It is useful to see where religious and secular positions overlap.

Asked by commission members to speak of Protestant and Jewish perspectives on cloning, Childress saw consensus for these religions (and for others too) in the belief that a child born through reproductive SCNT would still be "created in the image of God" and would have dignity. Consequently, people are obligated to reduce the harms to a child created in God's image. Beyond this, he recognized no single religious view. Roman Catholic thought, for example, regards reproductive cloning as inherently wrong, but Protestant and Jewish perspectives differ. Cloning is intrinsically wrong to some believers and not to others, who regard some uses as appropriate and others not. This justifies continued discussion as moral positions develop.

John M. Haas spoke from a Roman Catholic position. Humans have a "sublime dignity," he said, with rights and duties that are "universal and inviolable." Humans have a right to be born to parents in a "loving committed relationship," which is best served "only in and through the personal act of marital intercourse." According to church documents, medical science must not appropriate procreation, thus contradicting the dignity and the inalienable rights of the spouses and of the child to be born. Abdulazziz Sachedina spoke for an Islamic perspective, as he had done before the NBAC. He said Muslim scholars generally opposed reproductive cloning unless done to improve human life, but they did not necessarily oppose embryo research because they did not regard the embryo as a person. He expressed concerns about the impact of cloning on distributive justice.

The second set of witnesses dealt with ethical and moral issues. Ezekiel Emanuel, a bioethicist and member of the NBAC, reiterated Childress's comments about Dolly raising "unique and distinctive ethical issues" separate from those raised by embryo creation. Emanuel summarized arguments for and against cloning. Reproductive cloning is defensible for its grounding in two core American values: personal autonomy, which includes reproductive choice; and scientific inquiry, performed within ethical limits. Cloning is undermined, however, by the dangers it poses to offspring, a child's individuality, its attractiveness for persons who would clone themselves for vanity and treat children as products, and its potentially corrosive effect on family norms. Cloning warrants more reflection, he concluded, and the American public would not necessarily reach the same conclusions as a select group of bioethicists. In short, "ninety days is enough for a gut reaction, not a settled determination."

Edmund Pellegrino, a bioethicist, said the temporary ban recommended by NBAC and the president had two moral errors. First, something inherently wrong cannot be made right simply by the passage of time. Second, embryo research, which produces "death and dismemberment of embryos," is wrong and it is also the first step to cloning. The solution is permanently to ban cloning and human embryo research and to move on to more important priorities. Further debate will not necessarily lead to moral truths. On the contrary, continued debate yields to "verbosity, volubleness and verbiage."

John Robertson, a bioethicist and law professor, testified that sound policy requires more debate and analysis. Reproductive cloning may be defensible for couples who are infertile or at genetic risk. Moreover, the harms of cloning have not been carefully articulated, and cloning is "intimately involved with our freedom to make personal decisions about family and reproduction." He favored a voluntary moratorium on reproductive cloning and a more precise determination of harms, if any, in the meantime. He also favored expanding the debate to include inheritable genetic interventions.

The House Committee on Science scheduled a markup session to decide whether to report H.R. 922 favorably to the House. In anticipation of the markup session, Chair Morella convened a meeting of the Subcommittee on Technology for July 22, 1997. The original H.R. 922 had barred federal funds from research that would use "a human somatic cell to produce a human clone." The revised version would deny federal funding for cloning a human being *and* for research using "a somatic cell to produce an embryo." While the original H.S. 922 targeted the production of a human clone, the amended

H.R. 922 targeted the production of an embryo. Its broad definition of a somatic cell ("the cell of an embryo, fetus, child, or adult which will not become a sperm or egg cell") would encompass research into embryo and fetal as well as adult SCNT.

Following testimony from a biology professor and a member of a research association, two witnesses addressed policy orientations (U.S. House, CS-ST 1997c). A representative from the ASRM testi- fied that the association favored legislative restrictions on human cloning, but that embryo research was acceptable under controlled conditions. Any legislation to restrict reproductive cloning must be clear and precise. The ASRM proposed a narrower definition than that of H.R. 922:

[Cloning is] the duplication of an existing or previously existing human being by transferring the nucleus of a differentiated, somatic cell into an oocyte in which the nucleus has been removed, and im- planting the resulting product for gestation and subsequent birth.

This would not bar the creation of an embryo through SCNT, but it would forbid the transfer of that embryo to a woman's uterus. It would not restrict embryo cell or fetal cell nuclear transfer.

Alison Taunton-Rigby spoke on behalf of the BIO, an organization with 700 corporate members. BIO regarded human cloning as unac- ceptable but it advocated a voluntary moratorium rather than legisla- tion. If legislation is to be pursued, it must have a sunset provision, a research protection clause, and a stipulation that the federal law would preempt state regulatory laws. It must contain precise defini- tions. Taunton-Rigby brought a list of the varied definitions on the table from the NBAC, the administration, Ehlers, and Bond. Over- broad and vague definitions of cloning would chill research and not forewarn scientists about what was prohibited, she argued.

Taunton-Rigby thought Clinton's bill, crafted with guidance from the newly released NBAC report, was more sophisticated than H.R. 922, H.R. 923, and S. 368. Using Clinton's bill as a template, Taunton-Rigby proposed changes to make the bill more precise and congenial to researchers. Among other things, she recommended correcting the definition of SCNT, reconsidering "draconian penal- ties," and changing what would be forbidden. Clinton's bill would forbid SCNT "with the intent of introducing the product of that transfer into a woman's womb." She recommended deleting "intent," which cannot be implemented, and barring only the act of transferring the embryo.

Taunton-Rigby argued that several factors already constrained cloning: (1) the technological capacity to clone a person did not exist, (2) regulations in the FDA and NIH protected human research subjects, and (3) the voluntary moratorium would be effective if one looked to the "salutary example" of the long-standing moratorium on germ-line manipulations. She said H.R. 922 went beyond what NBAC and the president recommended, covered issues already addressed in existing embryo research law, and targeted embryo research more than reproductive cloning. Embryo research had already been "well-debated." If a law is to be enacted it should bar the use of federal funds for creating a human being through SCNT technology. This coincided with the ASRM's proposed wording.

Ehlers wondered why BIO used the administration's bill as a template given that the organization proposed so many changes to it. Taunton-Rigby answered that BIO used the most comprehensive bill as a starting point. The organization also thought the bill could be fixed. Ehlers pointed out that the two groups of witnesses had different bright lines: embryo generation or embryo implantation.

The ASRM and BIO representatives also observed a point made at the NBAC meetings: federal funding brings oversight opportunities with it. The absence of funding for IVF, they noted, pushed research to the private sector where Congress had no control over it. Were Congress to lift the funding ban on embryo research, studies would be conducted in public with review by peers, institutional review boards (IRBs), and the NIH. With the ban in place, research is not public and is difficult to monitor. The ethicist at the hearing had a similar concern but he reached a different conclusion. If the government neither funded cloning nor banned it, cloning would be pushed to the private sector. By implication, reproductive cloning should be banned altogether.

When someone at the hearing said the discussion was "drifting" when it turned to embryo research, Ehlers countered that the "issue of embryo research is very much here" and cannot be left off the table, thereby underscoring the key policy issue. Before adjourning, a committee member, Roscoe G. Bartlett (R-MD), sought agreement among panelists that the moratorium was working and there was a need to "enact the best legislation" rather than rushing to legislate.

The House Committee on Science met a week later, on July 29, to decide whether to report the bill favorably to the House (U.S. House, CS-ST 1997d). Subcommittee chair Morella said she could not support H.R. 922 because it was imprecise and could have deleterious effects on biomedical research and innovation. She said more time was needed to draft a consensus bill and that "not one scientific organization can endorse H.R. 922." Ehlers then moved to strike the text of the original H.R. 922 and introduce the substitute text he had mentioned at the July 22 hearing. The amended H.R. 922 barred the funding of research that would lead to the creation of an embryo through SCNT. It would also have the National Research Council study the law's impact and make recommendations for change, if any, within five years of the law's passage.

Immediately after Ehlers proposed the amended H.R. 922, Lynn Rivers (D-MI) offered an amendment to revert to the original intent of barring funds for the creation of human clones, not embryos. Rivers' amendment would forbid funds for the "creation of a human being using [SCNT] technology." This complemented the language proposed by the ASRM, an organization that had sent letters to committee members urging them to support Rivers' amendment with its more precise language. She said her amendment would bring consistency among the bills; the positions of the NBAC, BIO, and ASRM; and the funding ban already in place. Rivers' amendment failed, however, by a voice vote.

Rivers then moved to add a research protection clause to H.R. 922. The motion, passed by unanimous voice vote, added the following to the amended H.R. 922:

> The Act shall not restrict the important and promising work not specifically prohibited by the Act including the use of somatic cell nuclear transfer or other cloning technologies to clone molecules, DNA, cells other than human embryo cells, or tissues or the use of somatic cell nuclear transfer techniques to create animals other than humans.

Rivers expressed concern that the revised H.R. 922 "unnecessarily embroils the Committee in the controversy around human embryo research." She noted that the NBAC had avoided that controversy, as had the president. She was concerned that the ban on funding would be permanent, in contrast to the year-by-year appropriations measures that currently barred funding for embryo research. With a di-

TABLE 3.3 Key Policy Options in 1997

Proscription	Barring Funding	Barring the Act
Generating human beings through reproductive SCNT	I S. 368; original H.R. 922	II NBAC recommendation; Clinton proposal H. Doc. 105-97; H.R. 923
Generating human embryos through reproductive SCNT	III H.R. 922, as amended and voted out of committee	IV —

vided voice vote and barely a quorum, the committee voted to report H.R. 922, as amended, to the House. The meeting had taken less than an hour. Meanwhile, the president's bill did not gain a sponsor in Congress and no hearings were held on H.R. 923 or S. 368. Following the Committee on Science vote, H.R. 922 was sent to the Committee on Commerce, which did not convene hearings. The committee vote on H.R. 922 brought legislative activity on cloning to a close for 1997, with four primary policy options on the floor (see Table 3.3).

CONCLUSIONS

Lawmakers in 1997 agreed that cloning a human being was ethically problematic and should not be pursued, at least at present and possibly not ever. This consensus surfaced in the Congress, NBAC, administration, professional associations, and public commentary. Deliberations among academics, the public, and lawmakers focused on the type of cloning that produced Dolly, reproductive SCNT using adult somatic cells. Scientists used embryo cell nuclear transfer, fetal SCNT, and blastomere separation to replicate genomes in animals, but the ethical implications of these methods were not part of the debate over human reproductive cloning. Thus, whatever consensus there was related to reproductive SCNT.

For the most part, lawmakers took a cautious path in gathering information and exploring issues. The NBAC spent hours in public meetings and private interchanges weighing issues and writing a report. Both chambers of Congress held public hearings at which numerous expert witnesses representing science, bioethics, industry, and the law testified, submitted written statements, and fielded questions. In contrast to some European countries, where cloning had been banned, usually in connection with national laws on assisted reproductive technologies, lawmakers in the United States were in no hurry to regulate. While the NBAC grappled with novel issues raised by reproductive SCNT, legislators tied the debate to issues raised by embryo research.

By mid-1997, policy options revolved around several key questions. First, what should be proscribed—creating a human being through SCNT or creating a human embryo through SCNT? Second, what form should the proscription take—denying funding or creating an illegal act? Third, for how long should the proscription be in effect—temporarily or permanently? By the end of the year, as Sen. Frist put it, "cloning pretty much faded from the mental radar screen of most Americans" (*Cong. Rec.* 1998, S320). The administration had asserted its reservations and it set in motion a process to identify issues raised by reproductive SCNT. Professional associations representing the scientific community had pledged to honor a moratorium on the cloning of human beings. Technical obstacles indicated that reproductive cloning was not on the near horizon even if someone wanted to clone a human. It had taken nearly 300 attempts to produce Dolly, who by August 1997, was the only mammal generated with the help of SCNT and whose origins had not yet been verified. No reputable scientists indicated a desire to attempt human cloning. On the contrary, scientists were more interested in using nuclear transfer in commercial biotechnology.

CHAPTER 4

THE POLITICS OF REPRODUCTIVE SOMATIC CELL NUCLEAR TRANSFER, 1998

During congressional hearings in 1997, legislators periodically worried about "rogue scientists" who might ignore the moratorium and attempt to clone a human being. On January 6, 1998, the feared rogue took physical shape in the form of Richard Seed, a 69-year-old physicist without an institutional affiliation who announced on National Public Radio's *All Things Considered* that he would open a cloning clinic in Chicago to clone a human and employ a small group of hand-selected physicians once he raised the necessary funds (Kolata 1998b; Kestenbaum 1998). Seed had announced this intention a month earlier at a conference on genetic technologies and the law at the Illinois Institute of Technology. Only reporters from regional newspapers and the *Washington Times* covered the conference and nothing came of his rambling statement (Kestenbaum 1998; Johnson 1998). The *Washington Post*, the *Chicago Tribune*, and other newspapers picked up the "All Things Considered" story, however.

Within days the media, as one editorialist put it, "helped Richard Seed scare the pants off everybody" (Johnson 1998, quoting John Kass).

Despite the fact that Seed had no credentials for cloning a human and the odds were slim that even a research team with impeccable credentials could clone a human with existing technology, Seed's comments provoked a reopening of the cloning debate, this time with a heightened sense of urgency. On January 10, in a regularly scheduled radio address, President Clinton reiterated that he wanted Congress to ban the cloning of human beings. He repeated this in his State of the Union address on January 27. With the renewed effort to restrict cloning by law came an intensified politics with a growing constituency.

ACTIVITIES IN THE SENATE

Sen. Ben Nighthorse Campbell (R-WY) was the first to offer new anticloning legislation in the Senate, and he did so on the same day as the president's State of the Union address. Campbell, a former rancher and jewelry maker, believed the federal government had a moral obligation to prohibit human cloning. His proposed S. 1574 would bar federal funds for any research designed to clone a human being or create a human embryo and it would make cloning a human being or conducting research to clone a human being or embryo unlawful and subject to a $5,000 civil fine (U.S. Senate 1998a).

Although S. 1574 was the first new bill to be introduced, it was quickly preempted by bills introduced by senior senators. On February 3, Sens. Bond and Dianne Feinstein (D-CA) each introduced legislation that for the first time positioned carefully crafted bills from both parties against each other. Sen. Bond's S. 1601, *Human Cloning Prohibition Act* (originally and the same as S. 1599), contrasted to the modest two-line bill (S. 368) he had introduced a year before (U.S. Senate 1998b). With S. 368, Bond had aimed to bar federal funds for research that would produce a cloned human being. With S. 1601, Bond aimed at making the creation of a human embryo through SCNT a criminal act with a ten-year prison sentence for violating the law. S. 1601 would amend Title 18 of the U.S. Code to make it unlawful for any person, private or public, to use "human somatic cell nuclear transfer technology." It would forbid importing an embryo generated by SCNT into the United States, and it conveyed a sense to Congress that the government would cooperate internationally to forbid SCNT to produce a human embryo. It would also establish a National Commission to Promote a National Dialogue on Bioethics in the Institute of Medicine to deliberate about cloning and other topics.

Bond felt a sense of urgency about legislation, arguing that Richard Seed "forces us to engage in an immediate debate on how far on the moral cliff we are willing to let science proceed" before imposing restraints. Looking to progress in animal cloning, Bond said we "no longer have the luxury of waiting around for this morally reprehensible act to occur." Sen. William Frist likewise said Seed and others had "forced us to confront our deficits" and ask where to draw the line. He appealed to his colleagues to "help us stop Dr. Seed dead in his tracks." Legislation "must be crafted very specifically with surgical precision, with laser-like precision." In S. 1601 that line would be drawn at the generation of embryos through SCNT. The bill responded to "serious ethical dilemmas associated with churning out human embryos as if they were products on an assembly line" (*Cong. Rec.* 1998, S322).

On the same day Sen. Bond introduced his bill, Sens. Feinstein and Kennedy introduced twin bills. The lead bill, S. 1602 (originally and the same as S. 1611), brought under one umbrella both funding and prohibition issues (U.S. Senate 1998c). The two senators had met with officials from the NBAC, NIH, DHHS, and FDA, and members of the ASRM and the BIO to construct S. 1602. The bill would amend the *Public Health Service Act* (PHSA) to forbid creating a human by SCNT and to bar federal funds for the act for a period of ten years. It would "prohibit any attempt to clone a human being using somatic cell nuclear transfer and . . . prohibit the use of Federal funds for such purposes." To ensure continued deliberation about cloning, the bill would extend the NBAC for ten years and require it to report within five years and ten years on the issues associated with SCNT. S. 1602 called for cooperation with other countries to enforce restrictions on cloning. Feinstein resisted the pressure for quick action, saying Seed's claims were "somewhat implausible" given the "rudimentary state of cloning technology." Seed had, however, "hit a nerve" (*Cong. Rec.* 1998, S323–24).

This bill was more stringent than Clinton's legislative proposal of 1997 in that it provided for a $1,000,000 fine for violation (Clinton proposed a $250,000 fine) and it extended the ban on cloning humans for ten years (Clinton proposed three to five years). When introducing S. 1602, Feinstein and Kennedy warned that carelessly crafted legislation would chill promising medical research. Congress must be "prudent and judicious" in drafting legislation. A ban on cloning technology in general rather than a ban on cloning human beings in particular would deprive citizens of "invaluable" medical research relating to cancer, diabetes, and other diseases. Kennedy warned that a "blunderbuss ban" could impair or even stop life-saving research and impose "needless suffering" of people globally. He urged legislators to do "what the American people want—ban the production of human beings by cloning" while allowing important research to proceed.

The perceived threat S. 1601 posed to medical research mobilized a constituency with interests other than protecting the embryo. Members of Congress all received letters, including one signed by over fifty medical and patient organizations that cautioned against "poorly crafted legislation" and that urged Congress to heed for itself the ethical standard for physicians, "first, do no harm" (*Cong. Rec.* 1998, S322–23).

Two days after S. 1601 and S. 1602 were introduced, Bond moved to proceed with S.1601 to the Senate floor, thinking he had the votes to pass the bill. If approved, his motion to proceed would bypass the committee and hearing process and move S. 1601 straight to the Senate floor for debate. Bond asked if there was objection to proceeding with S. 1601 and Feinstein objected. She then started a filibuster on the move to proceed.

Feinstein pointed out that S. 1601 and S. 1602 had been introduced fewer than forty-eight hours before. During those forty-eight hours letters had begun to "pour in." She wondered about the rush to vote on S. 1601, noting that "this is not renaming National Airport Ronald Reagan Airport." She introduced seven organized letters received, including a lengthy statement from the BIO, an organization representing biotechnology companies and centers. The letters signaled the start of a mobilization by science, biotechnology, and medical organizations that regarded S. 1601 and the move to bring it to a quick vote as inimical to scientific research. While the debate heretofore had revolved primarily around values raised by embryo research, the debate now began more distinctly to encompass values relating to scientific freedom and commercial interest as scientists, industrial organizations, and patient advocacy groups perceived threats from the broadly worded S. 1601.

In its statement, the BIO agreed with lawmakers that it would be unsafe and unethical to clone a human being. It endorsed the NBAC's recommendations and asserted that the FDA had authority to regulate cloning. It worried about the possibility that persons might serve a ten-year prison term for conducting research that was not related to cloning a human being. It pointed out the disparity between Bond's minimal bill in 1997 and his more restrictive bill this year.

Feinstein introduced a letter from the American Association for Cancer Research (AACR), a group self-identified as the "largest professional organization of cancer researchers in the world" with 14,000 members. The AACR called for a moratorium on legislation for at least forty-five days. The American Association for the Advancement of Science (AAAS), an organization with 145,000 members and 300 affiliated societies, sent a letter calling for caution, as did other organizations and associations. The American Psychological Association urged lawmakers to consider human behavior as a whole and not just to focus on techniques. The ASRM urged senators to go through "proper legislative channels" to craft a bill. The letters rejected human cloning but urged Congress to protect medically promising research.

Upon request, Feinstein yielded the floor to Bond so he could make an introductory statement about S. 1601, but only if she could regain the floor after Bond's statement. She did, she said, "have a very lengthy presentation to make and it is going to be quite involved," which signaled the filibuster. Where Feinstein asked why there was a rush to legislate, Bond said it was necessary to act swiftly because of the intentions of Richard Seed. Moreover, the issue had been adequately debated: "This is not a new debate." Bond and Sens. Judd Gregg (R-NH) and Frist had talked with pharmaceutical corporations, researchers, and patient groups to construct what they considered to be a narrowly crafted bill: "[W]e intend only to prohibit, by cloning, the creation of a human embryo."

Given back the floor, Feinstein spoke of the need to define terms. One can only have a cloned baby if an embryo is placed into a woman's uterus. Her bill would forbid this act. She asked again, "Why does this have to be done in forty-eight hours?" and wondered "how many people do we condemn to death" by halting the range of research that would be made illegal if S. 1601 were to pass. Next, Orrin Hatch (R-UT) urged the senators to be careful in enacting legislation without committee hearings, especially on a complicated matter. His position illustrated the cross-pressures facing some senators who sympathized with the substance of the bill but disagreed about the wisdom of going straight to the floor for a vote.

The debate to this point pertained to Bond's motion to bring S. 1601 to the floor. Feinstein's filibuster announced her intention to keep the debate going. Eventually, Majority Leader Trent Lott (R-MS) sent a motion to close the debate (file for cloture) on the motion to proceed to S. 1601, accompanied by the requisite signatures of sixteen senators who must sign a motion to close debate. If the motion received three-fifths of the members' votes (60), cloture would be invoked.

The vote on the move to invoke cloture on the motion to proceed with S. 1601 was scheduled for February 11, at 10:00 a.m., with the half hour immediately preceding the vote to be divided equally between the two Senate leaders or their designees. Before the vote, however, the Senate resumed debate on the cloture motion the day before the scheduled vote, Tuesday, February 10. This had given interested constituencies four days, including a weekend, to mobilize. During this time, biotechnology and biomedical professional associations, patient advocacy groups, and scientists had drafted letters with multiple signatures (*Cong. Rec.* 1998, S561–64).

Kennedy and the BIO had earlier alluded to the authority of the FDA to regulate human cloning. Now Kennedy introduced a letter from the FDA stating the agency had jurisdiction over experiments involving human cloning and that it would "ensure that such experimentation does not proceed until basic questions about safety are answered" (Smith Holston 1998). The FDA did not, however, have the authority to decide whether cloning should be prohibited.

Kennedy introduced a letter signed by seventy-one medical and scientific groups and organizations. Noting the "unparalleled" opportunities in biomedical research, the signatories urged Congress not to rush to judgment. The Pharmaceutical Research and Manufacturers of America (PhRMA) had sent a letter to all senators the day before, which was also introduced into the record. Neither PhRMA member companies nor their researchers favored human cloning, but they feared a law that would "foreclose a promising line of research." PhRMA pointed to the FDA's asserted authority. If a law were to be passed, it should ban cloning human beings, not particular technologies. A letter to the American Society for Cell Biology signed by sixty-seven Nobel laureates who had received Nobel Prizes in physiology or medicine, chemistry, economics, or physics was also introduced. It endorsed the NBAC's recommendation to ban human cloning and it urged Congress to not inadvertently "interfere with biomedical research that is critical to the understanding and eventual prevention of human disease."

According to Kennedy, more than 120 scientific and medical organizations had spoken out against the broad reach of S. 1601. "[T]his is one of the most important scientific and ethical issues of the twenty-first century," Kennedy said, and it was introduced to the Senate only a week before. In the few days between, the "telephones in many of our offices have been ringing off the hooks from scientists and physicians and patients across the country who are deeply concerned about the impact of this legislation." Cloning was important but laws should not be considered under this "accelerated and indefensible procedure." Kennedy warned that research might be lost:

> Scientists can't use the technology to try to grow cells to aid men and women dying of leukemia. They can't use it to grow new eye tissue to help those going blind from certain types of cell degeneration. They can't use it to grow new pancreas cells to cure diabetes. They can't use it to regenerate brain tissue to cure those with Parkinson's disease or Alzheimer's disease. They can't use it to grow spinal cord tissue to cure those who have been paralyzed in accidents or by war wounds.

Feinstein said there was nearly universal consensus that human reproductive cloning should be banned. She criticized S. 1601 for imposing a ten-year prison term on someone engaging in research that "someday will save lives and suffering" and she noted that the bill did not define terms. She wanted proper procedures to allow contributions in lawmaking from scientists, particularly to provide definitions so the senators would understand what they were doing. Rather than "ramrodding" this one week-old bill through, Congress should follow the "normal deliberative process" of committee referral and hearings. In the meantime, the FDA had stated its authority and scientific organizations had pledged to a voluntary moratorium.

Letters appealing to Congress to protect research were introduced to the record from, among other organizations, the American Cancer Society, American Heart Association, Cystic Fibrosis Foundation, American Association for Cancer Research, Inc., Juvenile Diabetes Foundation International, Resolve, National Coalition for Osteoporosis and Related Bone Diseases, Alliance for Aging Research, National Health Council, National Patient Advocate Foundation, California Biomedical Research Association, AIDS Action Council (cosigned by the Allergy and Asthma Network/Mothers of Asthmatics, Inc., Alliance for Aging Research, Alzheimer Aid Society, American Academy of Optometry, and American Academy of Pediatrics), BIO, University of California at San Francisco, Cato Institute, American Society for Biochemistry and Molecular Biology, Beckman Center, American Society of Human Genetics, American Society for Cell Biology, National Association for Biomedical Research, Federation of American Societies for Experimental Biology, University of California at San Diego, University of California at Oakland, PhRMA, Genentech, Inc., and Ligan Pharmaceuticals.

On February 11, the senators assembled at 9:30 a.m. for the scheduled thirty minutes of debate (*Cong. Rec.* 1998, S599–608). Feinstein divided her fifteen minutes among herself and Sens. Connie Mack (R-FL), Strom Thurmond (R-SC), and Kennedy, a bipartisan group of two Democrats and two Republicans. Feinstein told of the volume of letters received from medical groups, and pointed in particular to the American Cancer Society's caution to move slowly. She focused on the promise of research for preventing or treating human disease.

Sen. Mack had a history of repeated cancer in his family in which he had melanoma, his wife had breast cancer, and his daughter had cervical cancer. His brother died of melanoma, his father had esophageal cancer, and his mother had kidney cancer (Mack 1999). On the floor he appealed to his colleagues to let patients speak and to allow normal deliberative procedures in Congress. He told of the diagnosis of cancer of himself, his wife, and his daughter and of the deaths of his brother, mother, and father from cancer. He urged his colleagues to "vote no on cloture so we have an opportunity to hear from those patient groups that want to represent people like myself, represent families that have been affected like my family has been affected."

Feinstein told her colleagues that her husband, mother, father, mother-in-law, and father-in-law all died of cancer. She said, "I know in their last days how important research is to patients and how willing they are to try new things." Sen. Thurmond recalled that his daughter was diagnosed with diabetes at age eight. He supported stem cell research for diabetes and other diseases.

Sen. Bond shared his fifteen minutes with Sen. Frist. He urged the senators to vote yes on cloture so they could begin to debate cloning. Pointing to the recent lobbying, he said there had been a lot of "inflamed rhetoric by some of the big special interests, the likes of which I have not seen in my many years of public service." He expressed distrust of "rogue scientists" and big biotechnology companies that want to create human embryos by cloning. He expressed concern that if embryos could be created by SCNT but not transferred, embryos would be destroyed. Moreover, it would be difficult to monitor to ensure they were not transferred. He wanted to discuss questions of embryo research: "[O]ur opponents' bill calls for the creation, manipulation and destruction of human embryos for research purposes."

In quoting a letter from a biology professor who said S. 1601 would ban the creation of embryos for purposes "entirely unrelated to the aim of cloning a human being," Bond added, and "well it should." Using embryos to generate stem cells and then to discard them is more than a slippery slope, Bond said, it is a "sheer cliff."

About moving S. 1601 to the floor, Bond said there was no need to prolong the discussion. The issue "is not going to be any clearer three months from now, six months from now than it is now." The only thing different will be that the "rogue scientist in Chicago" or others will already be trying to clone embryos by SCNT. Frist then argued that the bill's reach was narrow. "Do we eliminate all embryo research? No, only a single technique. . . . Do we eliminate all of this technique? . . . Absolutely not. . . . The animal research continues in somatic cell nuclear transfer." He continued, saying that science has been abused in the past: "We can look back at Hitler and what Hitler did in the name of science." He asserted that public involvement is needed and it can come from the commission proposed in S. 1601.

Other senators then took the floor. Sen. Hatch said he would vote yes because he wanted to get the matter to the floor for discussion, but he urged senators to be careful about intruding on research. Slade Gorton (R-WA) also would vote yes in order to bring the matter to debate. Harry Byrd (D-WV) would vote no in order to follow procedures and invite testimony from experts in congressional hearings. Richard Durbin (D-IL) cautioned against rushing to judgment. Kennedy said he could not let the comparison between Hitler and science stand on the floor without comment. Bond's last appeal was, "If you vote against cloture, you are saying yes to human cloning."

The senators voted on the motion to invoke cloture at 10:02 a.m. Forty-two senators voted to invoke cloture and fifty-four voted against. Four did not vote. This left the cloture motion eighteen short of passage. Republicans split their vote; twelve Republicans voted with forty-two Democrats not to invoke cloture. All voting Democrats voted against the motion; two Democrats did not vote. The vote meant that S. 1601 would not go directly to the floor, but would go through the committee and hearing process or be dropped. The vote was not a good litmus test for beliefs about cloning because the procedural issue split the vote. Lott withdrew S. 1601, although it could be resurrected at any time. This had turned out to be a sparring match involving the politics of embryo research and the politics of biomedical research (Rovner 1998). The bold politics contrasted with the more cloning-related deliberations of NBAC meetings and congressional hearings in 1997.

A HOUSE HEARING

One day after the cloture vote, the House Subcommittee on Health and Environment of the Committee on Commerce held a previously scheduled hearing to consider the ethical and legal issues associated with cloning (U.S. House, Committee on Commerce, Subcommittee on Health and Environment 1998). A diverse group of fifteen witnesses spoke, representing medical groups, religious perspectives, industry, and a cloning advocacy group. Subcommittee chair Michael Bilirakis (R-FL) wanted to explore cloning research that did not involve human embryos. He asked whether it was possible to reap medical benefits from the research without risking the cloning of human beings. Commerce Committee chair Thomas Bliley (R-VA) said that in the seventeen years he had been in the House, "Congress has rarely addressed an issue as important as the one we will discuss today."

Henry A. Waxman (D-CA) remembered how worries about r-DNA research were addressed without banning research or "micromanaging" science. To him, SCNT without producing children was not significantly different from ongoing genetic research. The FDA had asserted its authority over cloning. Legislators should avoid politics and find a reasonable way to approach fears in order to help "millions of patients." James C. Greenwood (R-PA) urged legislators to exert caution and to avoid "irrational or illogical assumption[s]." Fred Upton (R-MI) said the vote the day before was not close or partisan, but it did "[reflect] the caution and care" with which Congress should approach the issue. Frank Pallone (D-NJ) said in a written statement that the "prudent path" might be to codify the FDA's authority over cloning research. Greg Ganske (R-MI) wanted to discuss S. 1601 in light of potential medical benefits. Rep. Ehlers, accompanied by Sen. Frist, said the hearing was held to decide what should and should not be done. He wanted to forbid the cloning of human beings and embryos and he also wanted to protect research. Frist, too, wanted to protect science, but he wondered how much moral consideration should be given to the embryo.

The first panel of outside witnesses presented religious perspectives on cloning. A representative from the National Conference of Catholic Bishops regarded cloning as contrary to human dignity. A rabbi argued that knowledge was "value neutral" and the question was how to use that knowledge. Regulation, he thought, and not prohibition, was appropriate. A theology professor equated cloning with the manufacturing of human beings.

The second panel focused on science, technology, and ethics. A professor of medical ethics argued that the embryo was a human being, so cloning was unethical because it is "essentially human embryo research." A molecular geneticist who was also a Catholic priest testified that cloning would harm the human embryo and that SCNT is not justified "on human beings at any stage of development." A biology professor expressed concern about the impact of legislation on research, particularly that involving DNA transfer. She likened the issue to that of gun control. Congress may legislate the unethical use of guns but it may not take away the guns; similarly, Congress may legislate against unethical use of medical devices but may not take them away if they are to be used to promote health.

Two witnesses gave detailed analyses about what bills should look like if Congress regulates cloning. A representative of PhRMA said the association strongly supported the voluntary moratorium on cloning humans. While PhRMA did not believe legislation was necessary, it thought any legislation should focus on the act of cloning a human being rather than regulating an area of research. The legislation should include a clause protecting research, impose civil monetary penalties rather than criminal sanctions, protect researchers from lawsuits by individuals and groups, and include a sunset provision of perhaps five years.

A representative from the BIO thought it was a "bad idea" to transfer an embryo created from SCNT to a woman's uterus, and he believed this was the consensus in the scientific community. He questioned the need for legislation, especially in light of FDA oversight, but he urged caution if legislation were crafted. He mentioned the letter signed by dozens of organizations and sent to members of Congress in early February that had urged lawmakers not to do harm by prohibiting research that could help people with "deadly and debilitating disease." He included a lengthy written statement about the promise of stem cell technologies.

The BIO witness recounted the successful moratorium on human germ-line genetic applications, which was still in effect. The restraint shown by biomedical researchers in this area provided a "salutary example of the power of responsible, voluntary restraint." The BIO endorsed preventing human cloning by the moratorium on cloning humans and FDA oversight. The organization had informed its members about the moratorium and asked them to inform the BIO if they were conducting research inconsistent with it. When asked how long it would take to clone humans, he thought perhaps it would take one in a thousand attempts to yield a viable embryo. It would be hard to guess, he said, but this might take two to five years.

Witnesses representing diverse interests sat on the last panel. A representative from the American Association of Medical Colleges urged caution in legislation and said that "Congress has never legislated a ban on a scientific technology or an area of scientific inquiry." Doing so now could set a "very, very dangerous precedent." Legislation is a "blunt instrument," and legislation "driven by emotionality, misunderstanding and fear, tends to be very difficult to modify or repeal." He continued that "[t]o ban a nascent technology of such enormous potential benefit to our citizens and our economy solely for fear of a single odious application that has not even been proved possible would be tragic." It would be better, he said, to combine the moratorium with enforcement by the FDA or other agencies: "There is no crisis. There is no public emergency. There is no need to rush to legislate."

The chair of the Juvenile Diabetes Foundation International testified of the promise for research told of his daughter, who was diagnosed at eight years of age with diabetes, and of his personal interest in finding medical relief for this disease. The president of the National Organization of Rare Disorders was skeptical about the FDA's authority and questioned whether a court would uphold it. She proposed either enacting a narrow ban on cloning human beings or amending federal statutes to give the FDA explicit authority to oversee cloning technology.

The director of the Alliance for Aging Research spoke of the promise of research for "delaying and preventing" diseases associated with aging, including osteoporosis, stroke, depression, arthritis, Alzheimer's disease, diabetes, cancer, and heart disease. The last speaker, from Clone Rights United Front, read the Clone Bill of Rights: "Every person's DNA is his or her personal property. To have that DNA cloned into another extended life, is part and parcel of his or her right to control his or her own reproduction." He said that cloning would eliminate all infertility and that governmental interference in this area would be immoral and unconstitutional. He introduced a letter from an attorney who filed a constitutional challenge to California's anticloning law. The attorney wrote that politicians face only one question: "Who should decide whether and how an individual can have children? The individual or the government? Actually, it's a trick question. The Constitution permits only one answer."

CONCLUSIONS

During cloning's political resurgence in 1998, attention to reproductive SCNT diminished as subsidiary issues emerged. The general consensus was that reproductive SCNT should not be pursued at present, yet legislators made little progress in identifying issues raised by reproductive cloning. They did not explore the variants of cloning, including embryo and fetal cell nuclear transfer and blastomere separation. Nor did they reexamine safety issues in light of advances in animal cloning or ethical deliberations about such questions as whether one has the right to a unique genome.

The politics of cloning in 1998 expanded in breadth and gained in intensity so that medical and scientific groups seeking to protect research that was threatened by anticloning bills confronted pro-life groups who were seeking to limit cloning research. Interested persons with a stake in the policy outcome expanded in number and emotional involvement. Heretofore, the moral status of the human embryo provoked emotional, deeply felt values. Now research that promised medical therapies also elicited intense emotion, as the personal testimonies attested.

All of this indicated a subtle shift in the politics of embryo research. Traditionally, the potential beneficiaries of embryo research were a compact segment of the population interested in fertility treatment, preimplantation genetic diagnosis, and other reproductive technologies. The potential harms fell on human embryos and on society if embryos were treated as commodities and as means to other ends. In addition, the harm of not proceeding (lost knowledge) would be largely contained in populations with a stake in fertility treatment and reproductive research. The cloning bills provoked shifts in the perception of benefits and harms. The debates highlighted a growing group of potential beneficiaries of embryo research, namely, persons with debilitating diseases. The harm of not proceeding (lost knowledge) took on sharper form with the possibility that this would prolong the suffering of people with chronic diseases. Although it was unclear at that time how the research would help patients with disabling diseases and conditions, the mere prospect, combined with the threat of restrictive legislation, resurrected long-standing conflicts over embryo studies. The events of 1998 also showed the practical problems of crafting laws for a rapidly changing science, where changes in the techniques and uses of nuclear transfer rendered their definitions in legislative bills obsolete before the bills had even been voted on in Congress. In the meantime, various bills became more comprehensive rather than more numerous. For example, now all the options of Table 3.3 have been filled as S. 1601 barred the activity of cell IV, that is, the act of generating a human embryo through SCNT.

CHAPTER 5

THE POLITICS OF THERAPEUTIC SOMATIC CELL NUCLEAR TRANSFER, 1999

Those wary of anticloning legislation in 1998 warned that broad laws might limit promising medical research aimed at treating the diseases and debilitating conditions from which many citizens suffered. Testimonies of senators, letters from Nobel Prize winners, and warnings by industry groups all sounded a powerful voice, but in early 1998 their protests had to be taken at face value because they could only vaguely indicate what research would be hindered by broad legislation. By early 1999, however, scientists gave a clearer picture of potential therapies when they announced they had for the first time isolated and cultured human ES cells. This announcement catapulted cloning back into the policy arena, only this time with a difference. Now policymakers fit into their lexicon a new distinction between reproductive SCNT and therapeutic SCNT. With this distinction came new layers in the matter of a cloning policy.

THERAPEUTIC SOMATIC CELL
NUCLEAR TRANSFER

The fertilized egg, a single-cell entity also known as a zygote, is totipotent. From the Latin for *totus* ("entire"), the totipotent cell has the capacity to generate all the cells of the developing organism, including the extra-embryonic placenta (McKay 2000, 361). When the zygote divides into two cells, four cells, and so on, it becomes a cleaving embryo and later a blastocyst. While a blastocyst, the cells of the inner cell mass are pluripotent and have the capacity to generate all cells of the embryo itself except the extra-embryonic cells (McKay 2000, 361). Pluripotent cells are also known as ES cells: "[T]heir name evokes the stem of a plant from which leaves and flowers bud" (Buckingham 2000).

Over the years, researchers had isolated ES cells in mice (1981), sheep (1987), hamsters (1988), pigs (1990), rabbits (1993), rats, mink, and goats, and had described the ES cells of monkeys (Anderson 1999, 58–59; Wade 1998a). The isolation of human ES cells was elusive, however, so banner headlines greeted the news in late 1998 that James Thomson, a research veterinarian at the University of Wisconsin, had, in collaboration with researchers in Israel, isolated and cultured ES cells from human embryos donated by patients in IFV clinics (Thomson et al. 1998).

This news, along with the dual announcement that researchers had isolated embryonic germ (EG) cells from human fetuses, generated effusive speculation. Scientists predicted human ES cells, called "protean," "potent," "universal" cells, and the "mother of all cells," could pave the way for a revolution in medicine by producing cells for transplantation to patients with Parkinson's disease, Alzheimer's disease, diabetes, and other conditions and illnesses.

To isolate human ES cells, Thomson and his colleagues let donated embryos divide until they reached the blastocyst stage of approximately one hundred cells. At this stage, the blastocyst has a hollow sphere in the middle (blastocele), an outer layer of about seventy cells that have already committed to forming the placenta and other cell lines (trophectoderm), and a mass of about thirty undifferentiated cells pushed to one side (inner cell mass). The investigators removed cells from the inner cell mass of five embryos and cultured them in five separate cell lines. They froze four of the cell lines after they had divided for five or six months and let the fifth continue dividing. During the culture period, the ES cells retained their versatility and continued to proliferate.

ES cells are of interest partly because they are thought to have the capacity to divide indefinitely. Ordinary body cells have telomeres, or caps of DNA at the end of each chromosome, that shorten each time the cell divides until the cell eventually stops dividing. Cancer cells and ES cells are exceptions: Unlike regular body cells, they express telomerase, an enzyme that restores telomeres to their usual length (Wade 1998b). Thus ageless, they "never grow old" (Hall 2000, 33). While unlimited cell division in cancer cells is dysfunctional, in ES cells this trait holds therapeutic potential. During the brief time cells from the inner cell mass have ES cell properties, they can proliferate indefinitely in an undifferentiated state (AAAS 1999, 3). If they can be coaxed to differentiate, theoretically technicians can use ES cell lines to create large populations of muscle, pancreatic, and other specialized cells for transplantation.

The body at different stages of development produces categories of stem cells. ES cells are the most versatile; as pluripotent cells, they can give rise to all cell types, such as bone, muscle, and brain tissue. They can also produce gametes and all somatic cells and give rise to a functioning organism. Human EG cells are versatile but less so than ES cells. These come from the primordial cells of the six- to nine-week fetus and are the precursors of spermatozoa and ooctyes. They give rise to most cell types but not to a functioning organism. At the same time Thomson reported the isolation of human ES cells, investigators at Johns Hopkins University announced they had isolated human EG cells from aborted fetuses that had been donated for research (Shamblott et al. 1998). A third category of stem cells, adult stem (AS) cells, are multipotent cells, thought to be less easy to cultivate in culture and less versatile than ES or EG cells (NBAC 1999a, 9). AS cells repair and replace specialized cells, and they are located in mature tissue. For example, mesenchymal stem cells are located in tissue that supports bone marrow, and they differentiate to cartilage, muscle cells, and other cells to replace lost cells. Hematopoietic stem cells, located in bone marrow, help replace lost blood cells (AAAS 1999, 1–2). Mammals have approximately twenty major types of AS cells, such as those that can generate pancreas, bone, and liver tissues (McKay 2000, 363).

A tantalizing aspect of the prophecy about ES cells was the possibility of tailoring cells destined for transplantation to the recipient patient's genome so he or she would not immediately need to take antirejection drugs. The key lay in the nuclear transfer procedure. In one variant, an embryo would be created with an enucleated donor egg and the nucleus from one of the patient's somatic cells in a process similar to that used to create Dolly, but with a different intention (Solter and Gearhart 1999, 1469). When the inner cell mass developed in the six- to nine-day embryo, cells would be extracted and the embryo would be destroyed. The ES cells, now sharing the patient's genome, would be coaxed to differentiate to whatever cells the patient needed.

In a second method of therapeutic SCNT, technicians would transfer the nucleus from a patient's body cell to a previously obtained ES cell and derive a cell line from that (NBAC 1999a, 11). This, too, would customize ES cells with the patient's genome and eliminate the need for antirejection drugs. It would have the advantage of using existing cell lines without having to produce new embryos. Either variant of therapeutic SCNT would be a helpful but not essential part of ES cell therapies. With cells produced in the absence of therapeutic SCNT, the patient would simply receive antirejection drugs.

ETHICAL ISSUES AND POLICY OPTIONS

The isolation of human ES cells resurrected ethical and policy issues that had been a part of debates over embryo research since the 1970s and, more recently, of debates about reproductive cloning. ES cell research raised various questions about what research, if any, ought to be funded by the government and whether a distinction should be made between deriving and using ES cells. Further debate revolved around the source of embryos for ES cell derivation. Does it make a difference if ES cells are derived from spare and donated embryos from infertility treatment, from embryos created through fertilization, or from embryos created through SCNT?

Using Spare Embryos for
Embryonic Stem Cell Research

Individuals who accept embryo research in principle generally believe that the early-stage embryo does not share the same status as persons who have been born. These individuals accept studies on embryos, either in the early stage or by the fourteenth day after fertilization, if the studies are likely to advance the health of infants, children, or adults and if they adhere to certain conditions. As developed during the "golden age" of commission reports relating to embryo research and ARTs during the 1980s and early 1990s (Walters 1998, 339), it is expected that the research is conducted in a way that treats the embryo with respect. Among other things, researchers must use the smallest possible number of embryos, proceed only if the studies are likely to yield important information, and conduct no research beyond the fourteenth day after fertilization.

Those who regard embryo research as illicit, on the other hand, generally argue that the embryo has the same moral status as a person. Consequently, to use the embryo as a means for the good of others is to violate a principle that humans must be treated as ends in themselves. Opponents of embryo research argue that this principle holds true for the full life course, from the very beginning to the very end, including embryos, fetuses, neonates, persons in persistent vegetative states, and terminally ill individuals. To use embryos for research purposes is to treat them as commodities and to fail to give them the respect they deserve.

Those who regard embryo research as ethical generally agree it is acceptable to use spare, frozen embryos donated by couples in IVF programs who no longer need or want their embryos. If the embryos are going to be discarded in any event, it is argued they might as well be studied first, with the donors' consent, so that additional knowledge can accrue. Frozen embryos are not scarce; large numbers are in storage. In addition, it is argued that the disposition of the embryos is a private matter for their progenitors, who have authority over them and can use them for their own infertility treatment, discard them, donate them to other couples, or donate them for research.

Those who oppose embryo research respond that the destruction of embryos is a public, not private, matter because it involves moral issues of interest to all humans. They argue that couples can donate spare embryos to other couples rather than discard them, and they recommend producing fewer embryos in IVF clinics to reduce the number of embryos not needed by couples.

Creating Embryos through Fertilization for Embryonic Stem Cell Research

More contentious than the use of spare embryos is the matter of creating embryos solely for research with the sperm and eggs of donors. Those who support the creation of research embryos argue that some studies can be conducted only when embryos are created as part of the investigation. This applies particularly to studies aimed at advancing therapies for infertility. For example, the safe practice of intracytopolasmic sperm injection (ICSI), in which a single spermatozoan is manually injected into an egg, may become more reliable by testing the procedure on research gametes before clinical use. This will lead to the creation of research embryos, which will then be destroyed after they are examined to assess ICSI's safety. If the testing helps develop a safe and efficient ICSI procedure before clinical use, then in the long run more infertile couples may be able to conceive and fewer embryos will be lost in the process.

Another argument in support of embryo creation is that this will help avoid a skewing of research findings that may occur if research is conducted only on spare embryos from persons struggling with infertility. Regarding the derivation of ES cells, it is argued that creating embryos from donated gametes will enable the growth of cell lines from genetically diverse embryos. This will become more important as the time for clinical applications nears.

Those who oppose the creation of embryos for research argue that it reduces embryos to commodities and denies them the respect they deserve. Unlike research with spare embryos, where embryos are generated by prospective parents with the intent of starting a new life, here embryos are created with the intent to destroy them. This practice treats the embryo with disrespect and it may contribute to a societal hardening of attitudes toward embryos. Opponents also argue that there is no logical end to the process; once it is accepted that embryos can be created to benefit others, it is difficult to draw lines against subsequent—and possibly less important—studies. Those who criticize the creation of embryos for ES cell derivation regard the creation as unnecessary in light of the many frozen embryos available. They also argue that creating embryos for therapeutic uses may reduce the supply of eggs for fertility clinics.

Creating Embryos through Somatic Cell Nuclear Transfer for Embryonic Stem Cell Research

As described above, practitioners hope to combine SCNT with ES cell therapies to develop cells and tissues customized to fit the patient's genome. Here the idea is to use a patient's somatic cell to create an embryo that is genetically compatible with the patient. If ES cells are derived from the embryo, theoretically cells and tissues can be developed that will be compatible with the patient's genome and used to treat cells and tissues damaged by disease. Michael West, an advocate of therapeutic SCNT and later a member of the first research team to publish a study detailing the team's efforts to create human embryos through SCNT (Cibelli et al. 2001), sees the potential of this research. "What a dream," he has said, "to take a cell from a patient and take it back in this little time machine, of the egg cell, and make it young again" (quoted in Stolberg 2001b, A13).

Those who argue against the creation of embryos through SCNT express concern that this may increase the likelihood that SCNT will later be used for reproductive ends. Developing the techniques for successful embryo creation may prove to be too great a temptation, critics argue. To guard against reproductive SCNT, according to this perspective, no embryos should be created in the first place through nuclear transfer.

U.S. SENATE HEARINGS (1)

Talk of ES cell therapies in late 1998 revitalized the embryo research issue and created key policy questions. Heretofore, embryo research policy had taken the form of annual appropriations statutes in which Congress forbade federal funding for research involving the destruction of embryos. Under appropriations law in 1998, no federal money could be expended for:

> (1) the creation of a human embryo or embryos for research purposes; or (2) research in which a human embryo or embryos are destroyed, discarded or knowingly subjected to risk of injury or death greater

than that allowed for research on fetuses in utero under 45 CRF 46.208(a)(2) and section 498(b) of the Public Health Service Act (42 U.S.C. 289g[b]).

Would existing law allow funding for ES cell research? If not, should it be amended to permit funding for ES cell research? Showing the keen interest raised by ES cell issues, the Senate, NIH, and NBAC all convened meetings and hearings to weigh these policy questions. Although AS cells, EG cells, and ES cells were on the table, attention coalesced around ES cell studies.

Early exploratory action occurred in the U.S. Senate where a special subcommittee of the Committee on Appropriations held a three-part hearing on ES cell issues on December 2, 1998, January 12, 1999, and January 26, 1999. Sen. Arlen Specter convened the first part of the hearing to learn more about the isolation and culture of human ES cells that had been announced only two weeks before (U.S. Senate, CA-SLHERA 1999). Observers had already praised the studies for launching a "rich harvest of discovery" and for potentially bearing what one journalist called a "universal spare parts system" (Maddox 1998; Wade 1998a). The first set of witnesses offered abundant praise for ES cell potential. We know of "no biological limit to the numbers of these cells we can make," said James Thomson, whose team had isolated and cultured human ES cells. Harold Varmus, director of the NIH, predicted cell lines for almost every tissue of the human body could be generated in this "unprecedented scientific breakthrough." John Gearhart, whose team had isolated EG cells, and Michael West said ES cells would provide "enormous" medical benefits.

While testifying, Thomson and Gearhart described their work and argued that NIH funding was needed to realize the potential of stem cell therapies. With NIH funding, Thomson and West thought cell therapies would be available for Parkinson's disease in five to twelve years, and that the number of diseases treated would "increase exponentially." Later, Thomas B. Okarma from the Geron Corporation said NIH funding was "imperative, essential." Arthur L. Caplan, a bioethicist, said that without NIH involvement the "research will be driven solely by commercial practicality . . . and there will be very little accountability." Eric Meslin, executive director of the NBAC, said it was "absolutely essential." West explained the connection with

SCNT: If cell therapies combined with SCNT, patients would be their own cell donors. On the other hand, Richard M. Doerflinger from the National Conference of Catholic Bishops said the experiments were "abuses" and no money should be allocated to help carry them out.

The second group of witnesses disagreed about the morality of using ES cells, although not enough to dampen the supportive atmosphere. Arguing in favor of public funding for ES cell research, Caplan said "judgment and virtues" were needed, not "moral absolutes." He proposed a moral framework for embryo research in which the embryo has moral status not because of what it is but because of what it is intended to become. An embryo has one moral status when generated by a couple in order to have a child, but it would have a different moral status if it were not to be used to generate a child. According to Caplan, judgments about the morality of embryo research should be made on a case-by-case basis, not on a preemptive ban on all embryo research. He argued that federal funding for human ES cell research should proceed openly and with accountability from an oversight body and with guiding principles.

Doerflinger spoke strongly against ES cell research. To remove ES cells from the inner cell mass of a human blastocyst, he said, would be like removing the "heart and lungs from an adult human." The result is the same: The embryo is a "whom" and it is "killed." It does not matter whether the embryo is alive for only a short time or if a cow egg is used or if the resulting embryo could not be born. At issue is a "one-celled entity with a human nucleus [that] begins, even for a brief time, to grow and develop as an early organism of the human species." To derive cells from such an entity is "fundamentally wrong," even if the goal is good. Moreover, creating embryos through SCNT for customized cell lines would be cloning; it would produce "living human embryos who genetically are the patient's identical twin sisters or brothers." Doerflinger urged that attention turn to alternative sources for stem cells. He said research funded by the government must be ethically acceptable to taxpayers. Medical benefits in a civilized society "must not come at the expense of human dignity."

The next witness defended the private sector's ability to monitor itself. Okarma told how the Geron Corporation, which funded Thomson's research, had set up an ethics advisory board (EAB) to advise the company on ethical issues raised by ES cell research. The EAB reached conclusions similar to those reached in the 1994 Human Embryo Research Policy report (Geron Ethics Advisory Board 1999). Among other things, the internal board advised that researchers should not clone humans or mix the ES cells of different humans or of humans with a different species to make a chimera. Okarma thought the FDA should be the government agency to monitor ES cell product development.

Members of Congress convened the hearing to consider whether the existing law cited below, which equates the embryo with an organism, would allow ES cell research:

> The term "human embryo or embryos" includes any organism, not protected as a human subject under 45 C.F.R. 46 . . . that is derived by fertilization, parthenogenesis, cloning, or any other means from one or more human gametes or human diploid cells (45 C.F.R. 208 [a][2]).

Given that a multicellular embryo is an organism, is an ES cell also an organism? If yes, research using ES cells could not be federally funded. If no, the study of ES cells arguably could be funded.

During the hearing, the witnesses agreed that ES cells were not organisms, but they disagreed about whether the law would allow ES cell funding. West said ES cells were not organisms because they would not, if cultured in a laboratory dish, become a human being if transferred to a woman's uterus. Varmus said they were not organisms, but he noted that the NIH was struggling with the issue. Thomson said, "[T]hey are not organisms and they are not embryos." To Okarma, they were not organisms because if the cells were transferred to a woman's uterus they "would not form a conceptus nor develop." Caplan said they were not organisms because they lacked the "capacity to become viable, independent, interrelated, functioning entities." Doerflinger agreed that they were not embryos, but he drew importance from the fact that they were derived from embryos, which were organisms.

The second part of the hearing was held on January 12, 1999 (U.S. Senate, CA-SLHERA 1999). In a short meeting, in which Sens. Specter and Tom Harkin (D-IA) were the only members of Congress present, witnesses included two government officials who spoke of legal questions, a pharmacology professor, a representative of the Juvenile Diabetes Association whose daughter had type-1 diabetes, and a person with Parkinson's disease who spoke of his fears and hopes for research.

The third part was held January 26, 1999, ten days after the NIH, as discussed below, interpreted the law to allow funding for projects using human ES cells (U.S. Senate, CA-SLHERA 1999). Varmus testified that NIH funding would promote open discussion, public oversight, improved recruitment of researchers, and public health benefits. He announced he had established a working group to develop rules for conducting ES cell research ethically and that the working group's report would be published in the *Federal Register* for public comment.

Doerflinger urged the NIH to support research into AS cells that would not rely on human embryos. Varmus was asked whether stem cells could be derived without destroying embryos. He said at that point they could not. When questioned about the nature of ES cells, he conceded that ES cells could aggregate and look like they are developing into an embryo, but he said it would be unethical to test whether they were capable of becoming an embryo. Doerflinger and Sen. Harkin were engaged in a heated exchange when Sen. Specter adjourned the hearing.

LEGAL INTERPRETATION BY THE NATIONAL INSTITUTES OF HEALTH

In the same time period that the Senate was holding hearings, Varmus asked the general counsel of the DHHS to offer a legal opinion on whether the NIH appropriations statute would allow funding for ES cell research. The reply of the general counsel, Harriet S. Rabb, reached Varmus on January 15 (Rabb 1999). Rabb concluded that the law would not permit funding of the derivation (removal) of ES cells from the blastocyst because that act would cause the embryo's destruction. Even if a method could be developed to remove ES cells without destroying the embryo, funding would not be permitted under the law because researchers would have to destroy this experimented-upon embryo rather than allow it safely to be transferred to a woman's uterus.

On the matter of studying ES cells that had previously been extracted, Rabb reached a different conclusion. Because the law did not define an organism, Rabb consulted a scientific dictionary, which defined an organism as an "individual constituted to carry out all life functions." Under this definition, cells are parts of organisms but not organisms themselves, with the exception of unicellular life, such as the amoeba. Similarly, ES cells are not organisms because they cannot develop into an individual performing all life functions. As cells rather than organisms, as commonly defined, ES cells are not embryos. Funding of research on ES cells is permissible so long as the funded researcher does not actually extract the cells. In practical terms, this means researchers who secure ES cells from private sources may study them under federally funded research, but costs to secure the cell lines could not be covered by federal funds.

Rabb's office also interpreted the law relating to EG cells from aborted fetuses. The office interpreted the law to allow both the derivation and use of EG cells from aborted fetuses if proper procedures were followed. According to federal law, fetal tissue cannot be sold, the donor of the tissue cannot direct its use on a particular patient, the tissue must be secured under informed consent regulations, and the physician must describe how he or she secured consent and attest that he or she did not participate in the decision to terminate a pregnancy. In parallel fashion, she wrote, EG cells cannot be sold or directed to a particular patient, they must be secured by informed consent, and the decision to donate must be separate from the decision to terminate the pregnancy. The NIH position on the derivation and use of human EG and ES cells is summarized in Table 5.1. After receiving the interpretive memorandum, Varmus announced he would set up an advisory committee to develop guidelines for funding human ES cell research and that no funding would occur until the guidelines were in place.

With these questions, the difference between cloning bills introduced in 1997 and 1998, such as S. 1601 and S. 1602 become clearer.

TABLE 5.1 Legal Interpretation from NIH Office of the General Counsel

Type of Cells	Should Funding Be Allowed	
	For derivation of cells?	For use of cells?
EG cells	Yes	Yes
ES cells	No	Yes

Source: Rabb, Harriet S., General Counsel, Office of the Secretary, Department of Health and Human Services, Memorandum to Harold Varmus, Director, National Institutes of Health, 15 January 1999, photocopy (Andrea Bonnicksen, private collection, DeKalb, IL).

S. 1601 would make it illegal for any person to use "human somatic cell nuclear transfer technology," whereas S. 1602 would forbid the transfer of an embryo created through SCNT to a woman's uterus. The former would forbid both reproductive and therapeutic SCNT; the latter would forbid only reproductive SCNT. S. 1601 added a new element—it would make any form of SCNT illegal and subject to criminal penalty.

REPORT FROM THE NATIONAL BIOETHICS ADVISORY COMMISSION

On the heels of Thomson and Gearhart's ES and EG cell announcements, President Clinton learned that Advanced Cell Technology, Inc., had experimentally transferred human somatic cell nuclei to cow oocytes two years previously. "[D]eeply troubled" by the report of an "embryonic stem cell that is part human and part cow," Clinton asked the commissioners to consider the implications of research "involving the mingling of human and non-human species" at its November 17 scheduled meeting (Clinton 1998). He also asked the NBAC to conduct a "thorough review" of issues raised by human stem cell research. With this charge, the NBAC joined the Senate and NIH as bodies reviewing the ethical and policy implications of stem cell inquiries.

The NBAC dealt with the cow oocyte request first and expeditiously. Meeting in Miami shortly after receiving Clinton's letter, the NBAC consulted an embryologist by telephone and talked in person with the chief executive officer of the company that had conducted the cow egg study in 1995, who arrived uninvited (Hall 2000, 74). The NBAC members posed three questions: (1) If a human cell fused with an animal egg were transferred to a woman's uterus, would it develop into a child? (2) Would the product of a fusion of a human nucleus and an animal egg be an embryo? (3) If the entity were not an embryo, what ethical issues would its creation raise?

The NBAC responded with a letter to Clinton addressing each question in turn. First, it was too early to tell if the entity could develop into a child, but such an outcome would raise profound ethical issues and should not be permitted. The NBAC's cloning report had recommended against generating a child through SCNT, and this also precluded generating a child through SCNT with an animal oocyte. Second, it was too early to say whether the entity would be an embryo, but the issues would be greatly magnified if it were. Third, if the entity were not an embryo, its creation would raise no new ethical issues and the study would be akin to routine research (Shapiro 1998).

The ES cell issue required considerably more attention. Although in the middle of two other projects, the NBAC set aside time at seven meetings to bring in thirty speakers representing science, industry, medicine, ethics, law, and religion to speak about stem cell issues and to commission ten background papers. Some of the speakers had addressed the NBAC on cloning and others had testified in congressional hearings about cloning or ES cell issues.

The NBAC's recommendations differed from the NIH recommendations in one important respect: The NBAC would allow funding for both the derivation and use of ES and EG cells (see Table 5.2). While it did not recommend lifting the funding ban for embryo research, it recommended creating an exception in the ban to allow the derivation and use of ES cells from blastocysts donated by couples at IVF clinics (NBAC 1999a). It did not recommend funding at this time for embryos created for the research or for embryos created through SCNT.

The NBAC found "widespread agreement that human embryos deserve respect as a form of human life," but it found differences about what constituted respect. At the least, embryos must not be bought or sold and they should be used only for important research, when necessary, and when alternative cell sources are also pursued (U.S. Senate, CA-SLHERA 2000a, 15). The NBAC recommended funding for the derivation and use of ES cells because separating the

---

TABLE 5.2 Recommendations Regarding ES and EG Research Funding by NBAC

Type of Cells	Should Funding Be Allowed	
	For derivation of cells?	For use of cells?
EG cells	Yes	Yes
ES cells	Yes	Yes

Source: Rabb, Harriet S., General Counsel, Office of the Secretary, Department of Health and Human Services, Memorandum to Harold Varmus, Director, National Institutes of Health, 15 January 1999, photocopy (Andrea Bonnicksen, private collection, DeKalb, IL).

activities would interfere with scientific knowledge: (1) investigators would not be able to learn from the derivation itself, (2) if ES cells are not stable in culture, investigators could derive more ES cells more easily if they controlled the entire process, and (3) funding the use would limit derivation to only a few settings and might exclude academic institutions. The NBAC reached the same conclusion as the NIH legal counsel on EG cell research: namely, that both the derivation and use of EG cells were ethically and legally acceptable.

The NBAC based its conclusions about derivation and use on the ethical principles of beneficence (promote good) and nonmaleficence (do no harm). Withholding funding from the derivation and use of ES cells would interfere with efforts to heal, prevent disease, and conduct research, which would violate these principles. The research must be carried out with special care to ensure that couples who do-nate embryos give truly informed consent. As such, the NBAC listed things that must be told to couples in the consent process, including the following:

- the research will not benefit the couple directly
- the couple's future treatment will not be affected by their decision to donate or not to donate
- the research will lead to the embryo's destruction
- the embryo will not be transferred to a woman's uterus for pregnancy
- donors will not be able to direct the recipients of cells derived from their embryos (NBAC 1999a, 72).

To implement funding of EG and ES cell research, the NBAC pro-posed setting up a five-year National Stem Cell Oversight and Review Panel (NSCORP) to oversee ES cell use. The panel would review re-search proposals after IRBs reviewed them for compliance with human subjects regulations. In addition, the panel would do the following:

- certify ES and EG cell lines from approved protocols
- maintain a public registry of the protocols and cell lines
- compile a database of funded projects and those voluntarily submit-ted by privately funded researchers
- track the history and use of cell lines for future policy development
- submit annual reports to the DHHS (NBAC 1999a, 76).

At the end of five years, policymakers would assess research to date for benefits and to see if enough ES cells were produced using spare embryos from IVF.

According to the NBAC, funding was critical for public oversight and tracking of the research and to ensure that researchers protected embryo donors. The NBAC also proposed an incentive for privately funded investigators to submit their protocols for NSCORP review. If private researchers want to make cell lines available to federally funded researchers they would have to show the cell lines were derived according to federal protocol. The NBAC strongly encouraged private researchers to share their protocols with the public registry and voluntarily to adopt the NBAC guidelines. To guide private researchers whose projects were ineligible for federal funding (e.g., those using embryos created for research), the NBAC strongly encouraged professional societies to develop ethical standards and guidelines consistent with those recommended by the NBAC.

In recommending funding for both derivation and use, the NBAC found itself politically isolated. It issued a draft report with its recommendation in late May, affirmed this with a straw vote in June, released its executive summary in July, and produced its final report in October (NBAC 1999a). The Clinton administration distanced itself from the NBAC early in this process and allied itself with the NIH position.

NATIONAL INSTITUTES OF HEALTH ADVISORY COMMITTEE

Upon receiving the legal interpretation of the DHHS general counsel, Varmus had said ES cell research would not proceed until an advisory committee to be appointed by him had issued a report and opened it to public comment. The process began smoothly enough, as Varmus appointed a working group of the Advisory Committee to the NIH director. The working group met in April for a one-day public meeting, featuring as speakers representatives from the American Society for Cell Biology, National Conference of Catholic Bishops, Society for Developmental Biology, Alliance for Aging Research, House Pro-Life Caucus, and the NBAC. It completed its draft report in mid-1999 and released it for public comment in the *Federal Register* on December 2, 1999 (NIH 1999).

Following the guidance of the NIH general counsel, the working group set forth conditions under which funding for ES cell projects could commence. For procedures, it recommended that, in securing informed consent to donate embryos, investigators must (1) use only spare embryos from IVF clinics, (2) remove identifying information, and (3) ensure the donor couple makes one decision not to use the embryos and a separate decision to donate the embryos for research. The group recommended that the NIH set up the Human Pluripotent Stem Cell Review Group to oversee the research.

The group also targeted several areas of research that would be ineligible for federal funding, including:

- deriving ES cells
- using ES cells to create an embryo with ES cells from different individuals
- combining human ES cells with animal embryos
- using ES cells to clone a human
- using ES cells that had been derived using SCNT
- using ES cells derived in research using SCNT
- using ES cells from embryos created for research purposes

The public was given two months to respond to the advisory group's report. By this time, as discussed below, the politics of ES cell research had escalated. In view of the resistance by pro-life groups and the lack of consensus about the ethical acceptability of the research, the original deadline for public response was extended to February 22, 2000. In all, the NIH received over 50,000 responses. It revisited the draft guidelines in light of the public comments and released a corrected version of them in the November 21, 2000 issue of the *Federal Register* (NIH 2000). The NIH appointed a review group and solicited research proposals with a due date that was later extended to March 15, 2001.

THE POLITICS OF EMBRYONIC STEM CELL RESEARCH

Throughout 1999, ES cell politics were heated and persistent. Galvanized by Rabb's interpretive letter in January 1999, NBAC's open deliberations in the spring and summer, and the NIH Advisory Group's report, opponents inside and outside of Congress employed a variety of letter writing and coalition tactics, to which proponents responded in kind.

In early February, the Pro-Life Caucus of the House of Representatives sent a letter of protest signed by sixty-two Republicans and eight Democrats to Donna Shalala, DHHS secretary (Dickey et al. 1999). The signatories objected "in the strongest possible terms" to Rabb's memorandum to allow the funding of ES cell use, and they called on Shalala to correct Rabb's legal interpretation and reverse Varmus's decision. Jay Dickey (R-AK), the member of Congress who originated the NIH appropriations restriction on embryo research in 1995, and his co-signers argued that funding the research would "violate both the letter and spirit of the federal law banning federal support for research in which human embryos are harmed or destroyed." In the letter, Dickey said that federal law has protected human embryos for twenty years from "harmful experimentation at the hands of the Federal government" and has "provided a bulwark against government's misuse and exploitation of human beings in the name of medical progress." The NIH interpretation represented a change in the "ethical standard." Moreover, he wrote, Rabb had used a definition of the embryo (an entity capable of becoming a born human being) not supported in the law.

In the Senate, seven pro-life Republican senators, with Sam Brownback as the lead signatory, sent a similar letter to Shalala the next day expressing concern about a "unilateral attempt" to undermine congressional intent in its ban on funding embryo research (Brownback et al. 1999). They noted that Varmus had acknowledged in congressional hearings that ES cells could potentially start to develop as an embryo but that it would be unethical to test whether the ES cells were totipotent. The signatories argued that if one could not determine whether ES cells could develop into embryos it would be prudent to "err on the side of preserving congressional intent than destroying it."

In response to the House letter, Shalala asserted that ES cell research would be done cautiously and the NIH would proceed only with rigorous guidelines in place (Shalala 1999). Shalala said that Rabb correctly used the statutory definition of the embryo as "any organism . . . that is derived . . . from one or more human gametes or diploid cells." The law relates to research, she added, in which "'a human embryo or embryos *are* destroyed,'" not research preceding or following the destruction of an embryo.

On the matter of whether ES cells could develop into an embryo, Shalala wrote that mouse pluripotent stem cells sometimes formed an aggregated structure termed an "embroid body," which was not an embryo. Human ES cells could form embryoid bodies but they would not be embryos. Repeating that the research is "both legal and appropriate," she wrote that she respected the "deep convictions" of those in and outside of Congress about the matter.

While pro-life forces mobilized in opposition to ES cell funding, scientists and representatives of patient advocacy groups marshaled in support of the funding. Paul Berg of Stanford University organized the sending of a letter signed by thirty-three scientists from the American Society for Cell Biology to the president and members of Congress to support the NIH decision (Hubel et al. 1999). The signatories wrote that what they called pluripotent stem cells "cannot become a human being nor can they undergo embryological development." If the research is not funded, they continued, the nation's "most prominent researchers" whose work is supported by the NIH and National Science Foundation, will not engage in this research. As a consequence, advances will take place in the private commercial sector, away from public purview. With funding, on the other hand, research would proceed with peer review of proposals and heightened responsibility. The promise of this research for treating human disease creates a "moral imperative" to proceed.

Two weeks later, fifty-seven members of the House responded to Shalala's letter, saying the interpretation misstated federal law forbidding funding for "research in which" embryos are destroyed or discarded (Smith et al. 1999). The DHHS position was "less a good-faith interpretation of the law than an attempted end-run by those who have always opposed the law." Rabb's definition of the embryo revealed to them that "virtually no one considers the human embryo to actually *be* a living human being." To them, "a human embryo has no need to 'develop into' a human being because it already is a human being."

A week later *Science* published a letter from Nobel laureates and other prominent scientists who responded to the letter from the seventy members of Congress (Lanza et al. 1999). The signatories praised Varmus's decision as "laudable and forward-thinking," and surmised that ES cell research held "enormous" implications for medicine and for reducing the number of animal studies and clinical trials needed to develop and test drugs.

In the meantime, other scientific and professional groups developed documents for ES cell deliberations. For instance, the AAAS and the Institute for Civil Society (ICS) developed an AAAS/ICS position paper concluding that ES cell research did not raise novel ethical and policy issues (AAAS 1999). It recommended that the federal government should fund the use but not derivation of ES cells at present, a position similar to that of the NIH. Federal funding of ES cell studies was the most realistic way of committing funds to realize the promise of ES cell research. The AAAS/ICS paper did not call for a new regulatory body, saying that existing regulatory and professional oversight mechanisms would suffice with federal funding.

Throughout 1999, patient advocacy groups engaged in an active campaign to support ES cell inquiry. In one example, thirty-one nonprofit patient advocacy and research groups formed the Patients' CURe (Patients' Coalition for Urgent Research) in May 1999. This consortium's goal was to lobby members of Congress to fund stem cell research and to use patients' stories in the process. The coordinator later wrote that the coalition needed to "respect public sensibilities" while at the same time "court[ing] public approval fervently." In October, this consortium sent a letter supporting ES cell research to all members of Congress. Significantly, the letter was signed by four prominent theologians representing four religious perpectives: Protestant, Catholic, Judaic, and Islamic (Dorff et al. 1999). The authors agreed that in their religions "all human life must be protected." Yet they drew a distinction between different forms of human life. In particular, they distinguished between a spare frozen embryo that would not be used to create a child and an "unborn child who is already in the womb." The teachings of their religions stressed compassion, they wrote, and this extended to ES cell studies aimed at easing human suffering from disease. The authors believed federal funding and oversight would help ensure ethical conduct of the research.

On July 1, the Center for Bioethics and Human Dignity in Illinois (1999) released a letter signed by over three hundred people opposed to abortion and who condemned the NIH policy as "[i]mmoral, illegal, and unnecessary." In July 1999, Cardinal William Keeler of the

Secretariat of Pro-Life Activities at the National Conference of Catholic Bishops wrote a letter to the American Cancer Society (ACS) urging it to reconsider its affiliation with Patients' CURe. Then, shortly before a Relay for Life fund-raiser of the ACS, 100 participants withdrew from the activity (Wadman 1999) and the ACS announced it was withdrawing from Patients' CURe. The ACS later claimed it dropped out from the consortium because it was developing its own ES cell position, not because of political pressure. The ACS later developed a paper supporting funding ES cell research (*Nature* 1999c).

U.S. SENATE HEARINGS (2)

In light of the NIH legal opinion and the NIH Working Group's draft report, the Senate Subcommittee on Labor, Health and Human Services, and Education, and Related Agencies inserted a markup in appropriations legislation to allow research on ES cells if their derivation was conducted with private funds (U.S. Senate, CA-SLHERA 2000a). However, according to Sen. Specter, the Committee on Appropriations showed "strenuous opposition," as did some senators who threatened a filibuster. To avoid delaying the appropriations legislation, Majority Leader Trent Lott, committee chair Ted Stevens (R-AK), and subcommittee members agreed to delete the provision. They understood the matter would be introduced as a separate bill in early February 2000, when it would be more thoroughly aired (U.S. Senate, CA-SLHERA 2000a, 3).

Four witnesses testified at this hearing on November 4, 1999 (U.S. Senate, CA-SLHERA 2000a). Frank Young, a former commissioner of the FDA and now a minister, urged caution in moving ahead with ES cell research. He contended that "killing embryos by disintegration to harvest stem cells is illegal, immoral, and unnecessary" (U.S. Senate, CA-SLHERA 2000a, 7). He recommended that a fifteen-member, multidisciplinary commission be established for three years, with five members appointed by the president, five by the Senate, and five by the House to study stem cell issues. He called for a moratorium on ES cell research until the commission had done its work, and he looked to the FDA to consider whether new regulations were needed for IVF.

Dickey spoke next, saying that science should serve humans and not vice versa. He said the latter happened in Nazi Germany and in the Tuskegee syphilis study in the United States. He evinced concern that "our conscience is going to be numbed" if the goals of science mean human life is not treated with dignity. He said the distinction between the derivation and use of ES cells was duplicitous. "It is like being an accomplice to a crime. You cannot just sit there and watch something happen and then encourage it by receiving the goods from it and then say I am innocent" (U.S. Senate, CA-SLHERA 2000a, 13).

James Childress, a professor of religion and a member of the NBAC, next reported on the NBAC's deliberations and conclusions. Sen. Thurmond, a supporter of ES cell research, then spoke of his daughter's juvenile diabetes and of his many constituents who supported medical research. A written statement from Sen. Feinstein on the potential of ES cell research was inserted into the hearing transcript.

On January 31, 2000, Sens. Specter and Harkin introduced the expected bill, S. 2015, to allow funding for the derivation and use of ES cells from spare donated embryos (U.S. Senate 2000). The bill would essentially carve an exemption in the ban on embryo research funding. In relevant part, it would provide that:

> [T]he Secretary [of DHHS] may only conduct, support, or fund research on, or utilizing, human embryos for the purpose of generating embryonic stem cells in accordance with this section. . . . [T]he human embryonic stem cells involved shall be derived only from embryos that otherwise would be discarded [and] that have been donated from in-vitro fertilization clinics with the written informed consent of the progenitors.

In its other provisions, it stipulated that the research must not lead to the "reproductive cloning of a human being." IRBs would determine whether proposed research conformed with the NIH guidelines for ES cell research. This bill held both attraction and worry for scientists and researchers. On the one hand, it would allow funding for the derivation and use of human ES cells. On the other hand, it would enshrine into law a ban on all other embryo research, which had heretofore taken the form of an annual appropriations vote.

To prepare for the expected scheduling of the bill as a freestanding measure, a hearing was held on April 26, 2000, indicating the "very high priority" its sponsors placed on the matter (U.S. Senate, CA-SLHERA 2000b, 17). This hearing turned out to be the first of three held in 2000, and it foreshadowed the increasingly personalized political strategies of proponents and opponents. Frank Young, who had testified in the November 4, 1999, hearing, returned to testify against ES cell research, as did Sen. Brownback. Two scientists from the NIH (Gerald Fischbach and Allen M. Spiegel) testified in support of the research, as did two senators (Patty Murray [D-WA] and Harry Reid [D-NV]). Then Mary Jane Owen from the National Catholic Office for Persons with Disabilities told of her disabilities relating to vision and hearing and spinal impairments and of her reservations about ES cell research. While she favored AS cell research, she drew away from what she saw as a "frenzied pursuit based on fear" to cure disabilities and disease. She urged a different way of viewing disabilities, one that would accept disabilities as a normal part of life rather than as something to provoke great fear and lead to morally illicit research. "Do I want to see again?" she asked. "Do I want to hear as well as I used to? Do I want to dance again? Yes, it would be okay. But please know that I do not want those things at the cost of any living person. And I consider live embryos to be people" (U.S. Senate CA-SLHERA 2000b, 27).

Christopher Reeve, an actor and director who was paralyzed by a fall from a horse, testified about the potential of ES cell research for curing Parkinson's, multiple sclerosis, Alzheimer's, and other diseases and conditions. He noted that federal funding would ensure a wide dissemination of breakthroughs and allow careful monitoring of clinical trials. In a statement that stood in wide contrast to that of Mary Jane Owen, he said, "Again, why has the use of discarded embryos for research suddenly become such an issue? Is it more ethical for a woman to donate unused embryos that will never become human beings or to let them be tossed away as so much garbage when they could help save thousands of lives?" (U.S. Senate, CA-SLHERA 2000b, 38). The root of conflict over ES cell research—different views about the status of the human embryo—came through clearly among public speakers, just as it had among members of Congress. Reeve concluded his testimony by introducing the letter sent in 1999 by the Patients' CURe and signed by persons from four religions favoring research funding. He also introduced a list of numerous "disease groups, clinicians, foundations, universities and medical schools" also supporting ES cell research (U.S. Senate, CA-SLHERA 2000b, 41).

Jennifer Estess, an actress with amyotrophic lateral sclerosis (ALS), a progressive and ultimately fatal disease, next testified of the course of her disease and also of Project ALS, a group she had helped build of scientists seeking ways to replace neural cells destroyed by ALS. Lawrence Goldstein, a professor of pharmacology and an investigator with the Howard Hughes Medical Institute, testified in support of the research on behalf of the American Society for Cell Biology, an organization of more than 10,000 scientists. The hearing adjourned for a press conference that had been scheduled to cover the testimonies of Reeve and Estess.

The release of the NIH guidelines from its working group was delayed until August 25, 2000. Because S. 2015 was expected to be taken up on the Senate floor in September, the subcommittee convened its next stem cell hearing on September 7 (U.S. Senate, CA-SLHERA 2000b). Here only scientists testified. Two, Fischbach and Spiegel, returned from the April 26 hearing and spoke in favor of funding along the same lines as they did on April 26. Two others spoke in opposition. David A. Prentice, a professor of life sciences and co-founder of Do No Harm, Coalition of Americans for Research Ethics, predicted that ES cell research would devalue human life and set the stage for future disregard of individuals with life-threatening diseases. He spoke of the advances in and potential of AS cells as an alternative to ES cell work. Micheline M. Mathews-Roth, a medical professor, advocated AS and EG cells as alternatives to ES cell research. Speaking from a pro-life perspective, she called embryos "the youngest members of our species" and equated the extraction of ES cells with the tearing apart of the embryo (U.S. Senate, CA-SLHERA 2000b, 70).

The final hearing of the year took place on September 14, 2000 (U.S. Senate, CA-SLHERA 2000b). This time two scientists testified in favor of ES cell research, two individuals with disabilities testified in opposition, one scientist with a disease gave cautionary testimony, and four actors and actresses testified in support. Ron Heagy, founder of Life is an Attitude Foundation and a quadriplegic, opposed the research on moral grounds, and he spoke of the good quality of life that can occur after disability. Russell Saltzman, a minister with diabetes, offered that "if a cure for diabetes and a host of other ailments require the production and destruction of human embryos, then I beg you to consider the possibility that some diseases are better than their cure" (U.S. Senate, CA-SLHERA 2000b, 95). Anton-Lewis Usala, a scientist who also had diabetes, cautioned against future developments should ES cell research be pursued. Under questioning, he indicated concern about "science as an all-consuming fire" for new uses of embryos would be continually growing (U.S. Senate, CA-SLHERA 2000b, 102).

Jennifer Estess sounded a similar theme to that in her April testimony, and actress Gina Gershon spoke in support of Estess' connection to Project ALS. Mary Tyler Moore, international chair of the Juvenile Diabetes Foundation and herself a person with juvenile diabetes, spoke of the difficulties of the disease and of the hope offered by ES cell research. Michael J. Fox, an actor with Parkinson's disease, said he had watched the debate for two years, and he asked the senators to be attentive to the "real consequences" of the issue for people with diseases and not to "politicize a wonderful medical advance" (U.S. Senate, CA-SLHERA 2000b, 116).

On September 18, 2000, Sen. Lott tried to bring S. 2015 to the Senate floor. However, Sen. Brownback, using a particular rule, submitted an amendment to strike all but the enacting clause of S. 2015 and to insert an unrelated bill related to pain management (*Cong. Rec.* 2000, S9525; *Science* 2000). With that, the effort to introduce S. 2015 failed. It was reintroduced as S. 723 on April 5, 2001 (U.S. Senate 2001).

THE CHANGING POLITICS OF EMBRYO RESEARCH

The ES cell discoveries of 1998 contributed to a significant change in the landscape for cloning policy between 1997 and 2000. First, ES cell issues changed the constituency of those interested in embryo research and its applications. In the late 1970s and early 1980s, when IVF commenced, researchers envisioned embryo research primarily to improve infertility treatment, not to promote medical therapies for the broader population. There were numerous reasons for this. In part, it was a self-imposed limit relating to equity. If patients donated their gametes or spare embryos for research, the reasoning went, the community of those trying to conceive should reap the benefits. Even though the donors themselves would not benefit from increased knowledge, others in the same community might in the future. Embryo research would contribute to improved success IVF rates and refined infertility treatments. As early as 1979, the U.S. EAB foresaw ends of embryo research as primarily related to infertility and reproduction (DHEW, EAB 1979, 169–70). The British articulated this approach in the Warnock Report of 1984 and translated it to law with the 1990 *Human Fertilisation and Embryology Act* (Warnock 1985). Canada's Royal Commission on New Reproductive Technologies (1993, 613) likewise regarded research related to infertility causes and treatment as a high priority for research using human embryos. Although these and other commissions anticipated broader research ends in the future, including ES cell developments, these were not emphasized (see, e.g., DHEW, EAB 1979, 170; NIH 1994, 19–20).

Narrowly perceived ends of embryo research in the early years could also be traced to conflicts about the morality of the research. Even then, embryo research was a scientific pariah. The United Kingdom was the only nation that enabled these studies with any degree of support. Other nations either banned nontherapeutic interventions on embryos, explicitly withheld funding from them, or merely tolerated them through policy inaction. The wariness toward embryo research was apparent early in the United States, when the EAB recommended federal funding but was ignored and later disbanded. An additional effort to fund embryo research in 1994 likewise met with an immediate withdrawal of support when the HERP—convened to distinguish between ethically acceptable and unacceptable forms of embryo research—recommended, among other things, funding for projects in which embryos were created for research purposes. With governmental opposition, scientists evinced little interest in broader goals of embryo research, and research was on a minimal, ad hoc, and unmonitored basis. Prior to the late 1990s, clinicians, researchers, and patients lobbied without much hope of changing embryo research policy to permit governmental funding.

This resignation turned to action when reproductive SCNT rekindled an interest in embryo research issues and when congressional efforts to limit SCNT in 1997, 1998, and 1999 (and later 2001) threatened to bar a large swath of research. Talk of "universal" cells, a revolution in transplant medicine, and anti-aging interventions broadened the putative beneficiaries of embryo research. Among those who might gain from ES cell therapies were patients with debilitating diseases, persons who had relatives with chronic diseases or who worried they would themselves one day have these diseases, patient advocacy groups, health care professionals, biotechnology companies, and researchers. Several diseases were highlighted in particular, including Parkinson's disease, Alzheimer's disease, cancer, and diabetes. This propelled embryo research from the world of infertility treatment to the broader context of clinical medicine.

A second change came in the way costs and benefits of the research were framed. Heretofore in the public debate, the predicted costs of embryo research appeared to outweigh the benefits. Those opposed to the research held the political advantage in the United States. They, who included a large and passionate constituency, argued a moral position that the research would be an immoral destruction of human life for the benefit of others. This placed proponents in an awkward position of arguing for research that would, in pursuit of what they considered beneficial ends, destroy the embryos that were perceived by many groups as humans needing protection. While this was held by critics to be a significant moral affront, there was little on the benefit side to counterbalance the charge that scientists were killing embryos. The prospective benefits were largely confined to the fertility community, which in turn was relatively circumscribed. Moreover, lingering perceptions that infertility was not a disease and that treatment was a luxury rather than a necessity failed to elicit widespread public sympathy in support of the community. In addition, many inroads had been made in infertility treatment without systematic embryo research in the United States, making some think there was no need to start now.

The commentary accompanying ES cell discoveries shifted the cost-benefit paradigm to narrow the perceived costs and expand the potential benefit. Previously, with embryo research in general, the perception took root that unknown numbers of embryos would be destroyed for research. Now, one aspect of the ES cell debate highlighted the possibility that only a small number of embryos would be needed to produce an ample supply of ES cells for distribution to investigators. Moreover, proponents stressed that ES cell research would be limited to research on spare unwanted embryos that were going to be destroyed in any event.

If costs, in terms of embryo life, would be carefully limited with ES cell studies, the potential benefits were said to be exponential. They also were, if they took the form of medical therapies, tangible, in contrast to the costs, which were largely moral in nature. One witness in the stem cell hearings stated the perceived balance as follows:

> The embryos that are being discussed, according to science, bear as much resemblance to a human being as a goldfish. I think that makes the answer clear. We are dealing with flesh and blood people now who feel pain, feel fear, feel debilitation, and our obligation is to those who are here (U.S. Senate, CA-SLHERA 2000b, 118).

In addition, a new element in the calculation embraced the argued cost of *not* proceeding. Sen. Harkin warned in one of the 2000 stem cell hearings: "No one can guarantee what [stem cell research] is going to lead to, but to blindly stop it now or to tie one hand behind our back I think is basically to doom millions of Americans and people around the world to perhaps lives that they might not otherwise be leading" (U.S. Senate, CA-SLHERA 2000b, 14). In the same hearing, Sen. Specter said, "[T]here needs to be a sense of urgency to getting this done because every day is a day lost which could be saving lives" (U.S. Senate, CA-SLHERA 2000b, 17). In a later hearing, one investigator said, "[W]e believe it would be immoral not to pursue embryonic stem cell research, within the appropriate regulatory oversight mandated by the NIH Guidelines, because this research has enormous potential to save human lives and to mitigate human suffering" (U.S. Senate, CA-SLHERA 2000b, 86).

A third shift in the political climate lay in the increasingly refined and effective lobbying methods engaged in by both proponents and opponents. For one thing, both sides capitalized on unexpected positions taken by persons associated with disease. Proponents of ES cell funding pointed to pro-life individuals who supported ES cell research, such as Sen. Gordon Smith (R-OR), who had Parkinson's in his family and who wrote a letter to his constituents explaining his position: "My pro-life beliefs guide me to make life better for the living as well, to relieve suffering where there is pain, and to find cures for deadly diseases wherever possible" (Toner 2001). Proponents also referred to Sen. Thurmond's support of the research, which was apparently influenced by the conservative senator's experience with his daughter's juvenile diabetes. In another instance, two Republican senators, Thurmond and Brian Bilbray (R-CA), held a press conference endorsing ES cell research (Wadman 1999). The sponsorship by Sens. Harkin and Specter, a Democrat and Republican respectively, of S. 2015, and the advocacy of each senator in the stem cell hearings underscored the relatively unusual sight of bipartisan support. Months later, when the Republican administration of George W. Bush grappled with the ES cell issue, one official looked at mixed partisan alignments and said, "We're into new territory here. It doesn't slice nice" (Bruni 2001).

Opponents of ES cell funding pointed to persons with disabilities who opposed ES cell research, such as Mary Jane Owen, Ron Heagy, and Russell Saltzman, who were witnesses in the 2000 ES cell hearings. These and other witnesses expressed the view that there were alternatives to ES cell research that would be less morally problematic, and they made it clear their pro-life positions weighed more heavily than their hope of medical breakthroughs. In addition, each hearing generally included at least one scientist who opposed ES cell research.

The use of celebrities furthered the interests of supporters of ES cell research, and several formed their own research and lobbying organizations, including the Christopher Reeve Paralysis Foundation and the Michael J. Fox Foundation for Parkinson's Research. In pursuit of coalition building, scientists formed Do No Harm and other groups to oppose ES cell research. Nobel-prize-winning scientists signed letters of support. One of these, signed by eighty Nobel laureates in February 2001, was held to be the "biggest collection of Nobel signatures ever sent to a president" (Weiss 2001). Other scientists and groups representing the interests of persons with diseases also signed petitions, such as a letter signed by over a hundred groups and introduced into the April 26, 2000, hearings.

The lucrative potential for therapies stemming from ES cell studies also changed the climate for cloning policy between 1997 and 2000. Fearing overly broad legislation, the BIO, Pharmaceutical Research and Manufacturers Association, and other organizations mobilized to protect manufacturers' interests. If corporations had not previously pursued embryo research because predicted financial paybacks did not outweigh political costs and negative publicity, the equation now shifted. Buoyed by a broadly supportive constituency and prospects for significant commercial gain, biotechnology companies and academic researchers proceeded with plans to pursue stem cell research. While some researchers focused on EG and AS as less problematic alternatives, others prepared to proceed with ES cells. James Thomson's institution, the University of Wisconsin, had retained its rights to distribute ES cells, and it set up an institute to distribute ES cell lines. Within a month of announcing it would begin distribution after federal guidelines were in place, it received 100 requests from private and public investigators for ES cell lines (Marshall 2000d, 1420).

Despite these developments, the shifting politics of embryo research did not result in any policy changes or in the enforcement of existing policy. By mid-2001, the NIH had not reviewed any ES cell proposals. In January 2001, the Democratic administration of Bill Clinton handed power to the Republican administration of George W. Bush. While the new DHHS secretary, Tommy G. Thompson, had openly supported ES cell research when he was governor of Wisconsin, he was circumspect about his position after taking the role of a cabinet member in an administration with a pro-life platform. A call for proposals had been released in late 2000 and the NIH had appointed a review group with plans to meet in April 2001. At the last minute, however, the DHHS issued an order to suspend the meeting. Next, religious organizations initiated a suit to halt federal funding of ES cell research. A judge temporarily postponed the suit until DHHS completed a new review of its own on whether it could fund ES cell research under the current law. In response to the suit, ES cell researchers, including James Thomson, John Gearhardt, and Alan Trounson, and three patient advocates, including Christopher Reeve, on May 8 filed a motion claiming the DHHS failure to implement the NIH guidelines harmed them and violated the *NIH Revitalization Act* (Aker 2001).

In the meantime, a global network, ESCellsInt-ESI, with members from nations including Singapore, the Netherlands, Israel, and the United States, was set up to make cell lines available worldwide to academic researchers (Aker 2001). Other sources of funding also emerged. For example, an anonymous grant of $58.5 million was given to the Johns Hopkins University School of Medicine to set up an Institute for Cell Engineering to fund ES and AS cell research

(Pulley 2001). Eventually, in late 2001, the administration opened limited ES cell research for federal funding. On August 9, 2001, in a nationally televised speech, President Bush announced that the government would consider funding ES cell research using cell lines that had previously been derived from embryos donated by couples in IVF clinics who no longer wanted or needed them for their conception efforts. Informed consent procedures were necessary and couples were not to have been offered "financial inducements" to donate (NIH, Office of the Director 2001a). The number of ES cell lines was later said to be sixty-seven at eleven institutions, many of them in other nations (*Science* 2001d). The NIH review group formed during the Clinton administration was disbanded (NIH, Office of the Director 2001b) and November 27, 2001, was set as the first deadline for the submission of grant proposals.

CONCLUSIONS

The stem cell politics underscored the deep divisions regarding embryo research that played out in predictable yet escalating ways, with hyperbolic as well as thoughtful arguments on both sides. In the shadow of the ES cell issue, reproductive cloning faded but was not lost. Although members of Congress introduced new bills to bar reproductive cloning, the difficulty of enacting legislation relating to embryos made the prospect of enacting laws to regulate human cloning elusive. Philosopher Alistair MacIntyre had once said about abortion, "I do not mean by this just that such debates go on and on and on—although they do—but also that they can apparently find no terminus. There seems to be no rational way of securing moral agreement in our culture" (NBAC 1999a, 51). Held to be the most contentious political issue of Bush's early months in office, ES cell questions underscored the political as well as the scientific complexity of the issue. ES cell research had the tendency to "scramble conventional notions of left and right" (Toner 2001) and make it difficult to predict whether legislation would be enacted. Whatever the outcome, an alternative approach for reproductive SCNT relying on existing regulatory mechanisms was also possible, as discussed in the next three chapters. Whatever the immediate outcome, a political change had taken place and was here to stay.

CHAPTER 6

ADMINISTRATIVE OVERSIGHT: FOOD AND DRUG ADMINISTRATION

When witnesses mentioned the FDA as a potential participant in cloning oversight in 1997, members of Congress took little note. When the idea arose again in 1998 and 1999, however, some members took the prospect more seriously, not the least because the FDA was the sole governmental agency that asserted immediate jurisdiction over reproductive SCNT. In the existing regulatory apparatus, the FDA plays a key role. What is the nature of FDA involvement in reproductive SCNT policy? How sufficient is it for innovative reproductive and genetic technologies in the future?

NATURE OF FOOD AND DRUG ADMINISTRATION OVERSIGHT

As part of its authority over medical products, the FDA regulates biologic products, drugs, and medical devices (see Table 6.1). Biologic products derive from living matter and drugs from chemical combi-

---

TABLE 6.1 Medical Products Regulated by the FDA

Drug
"[An article] intended for use in the diagnosis, cure, mitigation, treatment, or prevention of disease in man or other animals"

Device
"An instrument, apparatus, . . . or similar or related article . . . intended for use in the diagnosis of disease or other conditions, or in the cure, mitigation, treatment, or prevention of disease, in man or other animals . . . which does not achieve its primary intended purposes through chemical action within or on the body of man or other animals and which is not dependent upon being metabolized for the achievement of its primary intended purposes"

Biologic product
"A virus, therapeutic serum, toxin, antitoxin, vaccine, blood, blood component or derivative, allergenic product, analogous product, or arsphenamine or derivative of arsphenamine (or any other trivalent organic arsenic compound) applicable to the prevention, treatment, or cure of a disease or condition of a human being"

Source: Public Health and Safety Act, 21 U.S.C. 321.

nations. Medical devices are instruments that do not produce a chemical action in the body, such as pacemakers. Biologic products can take the form of manipulated cells or tissues, such as placing cells on biodegradable scaffolds to form tissue to replace missing or diseased tissues (Malinowski 2000, 219). To establish the FDA's role in therapeutic and reproductive SCNT, it is necessary to accept that ES cell therapies and embryos generated through SCNT are biologic products.

Through most of the twentieth century, biologic products (biologics) were a simple category that included blood products, vaccines, and allergenic extracts (Noguchi 1996, 368). However, changing technologies in the latter part of the century resulted in expanded definitions. Under today's law, a biologic is

> [a] virus, therapeutic serum, toxin, antitoxin, vaccine, blood, blood component or derivative, allergenic product, analogous product, or arsphenamine or derivative of arsphenamine (or any other trivalent organic arsenic compound) applicable to the prevention, treatment, or cure of a disease or condition of a human being (21 U.S.C. 321).

New biologics are regularly approved for marketing. For example, in 1997 the FDA approved fifteen biologics, including RabAvert, a rabies vaccine to immunize people against rabies before or after exposure; Remicade, designed to treat persons with moderate or severe Crohn's disease; and RotaShield, a vaccine to protect infants against rotavirus. It also approved seventeen new or expanded uses for existing products, such as Neupogen, approved for treating acute myeloid leukemia (DHHS, FDA, Center for Biologics Evaluation and Research [CBER] 1998).

Two parts of the definition admit considerable flexibility and, as seen below, play a role in cloning policy. First, the "analogous product," as interpreted by the FDA, is broad enough to include gene and ES cell therapies. Second, products must aim to prevent, treat, or cure a disease or "condition." The word "condition" was quietly added to the FDA's authority by Congress in the *Food and Drug Administration Modernization Act of 1997*, and it set the stage for therapies designed to remedy infertility (U.S. Senate, CLHS-SPHS 1997c, 161). Thus, if one accepts that an embryo created through SCNT is an "analogous product" designed to treat the "condition" of infertility, this establishes a statutory basis under the PHSA and the *Food, Drug and Cosmetic Act* for FDA oversight of reproductive SCNT. If one does not accept these interpretations, then the statutory basis for FDA oversight is open to challenge.

The U.S. government asserted authority over the marketing of biologics in the early twentieth century in response to deaths associated with dangerous products (Brody 2000, 676). In one instance, thirteen children died from tetanus after being inoculated with a contaminated diphtheria vaccine from a horse that had contracted tentaus (Noguchi 1996, 367). In response, Congress passed the *Biologics Control Act of 1902*, which required the government to regulate biologic products for safety, purity, and potency (Kessler et al. 1993). Among other things, biologics were to be prepared in licensed facilities so that their safety and purity could be ensured before they were marketed, and packaged drugs had to be labeled with a date and manufacturer's address (Noguchi 1996, 368). The *Biologics Control Act* is now codified as the PHSA (Merrill and Javitt 2000, 321).

In a second instance, in the 1930s one hundred children died after being given a drug that had been inadequately tested before reaching the market (Brody 2000, 676). In response, Congress passed the *Food,*

Drug, and Cosmetic Act of 1938 (FDCA), which required drug manu-facturers to show that drugs were safe before they could put the products on the market by completing a new drug application (NDA). Then, in the 1950s thousands of children outside the United States were born with missing or deformed limbs after their mothers took thalidomide for morning sickness while pregnant. Congress re-sponded in 1962 by requiring manufacturers to show the safety of drugs earlier than at the stage of marketing. Manufacturers now had to show evidence of safety before the product could be tested on human subjects. This added a new regulatory step in which manufac-turers had to complete an investigational new drug application (IND) before testing drugs on human subjects. Congress also stepped up the requirements for the NDA, requiring manufacturers to show in their NDA that the drug was effective as well as safe (Brody 2000, 676).

Congress gave responsibility for the regulation of biologics that are part of interstate commerce to the Public Health Service in 1944, and that responsibility was transferred to the FDA in 1972 (U.S. Sen-ate, CLHS-SPHS 1997c, 2, 39). The FDA's statutory authority de-rives primarily from the PHSA and from the FDCA of 1938, as re-vised in 1962, 1976, 1980, and 1997 (Merrill and Javitt 2000, 321). The agency has used its wide discretionary authority to modify its oversight procedures since 1972 (Brody 2000, 676).

FDA oversight technically begins when new drugs, devices, and bi-ologics in the process of development are first tested on human sub-jects, and it ends when the products are distributed in the market (Kessler et al. 1993). A biologic is regarded as new, and thereby sub-ject to oversight, if it is not generally recognized as safe and effective among medical experts. New drugs are regulated under the FDCA, and biologic products are subject to additional oversight under the PHSA (Malinowski 2000, 217). The FDCA focuses on safety and ef-ficacy of the product while the PHSA focuses on the manufacturing process (Malinowski 1999, 11.13).

Two centers in the FDA regulate products. The CBER regulates biologic products primarily under the PHSA, and the Center for Drug Evaluation and Research (CDER) regulates drugs under the FDCA (Malinowski 1999, 11.14). CBER and CDER follow similar procedures, although they have different organizational structures (U.S. Senate, CLHS-SPHS 1997c, 39). Over time, the agency has blended its oversight of drugs and biologics. The CBER is also authorized under Section 351 of the PHSA to prevent the transmission of communicable diseases among states and from other nations to the states (DHHS, FDA 1998, 2, 30, 7).

The FDA's authority over food, cosmetics, drugs, medical devices, and biologics reaches over a third of the products marketed in the United States. These products must be part of interstate commerce to create a federal jurisdiction. The Supreme Court has broadly interpreted interstate commerce (*Scarborough v. United States*, 431 US 563 [1997]), as has the FDA, which asserts that interstate commerce includes a product, component of a product, or patient with a product moving across state lines (NBAC 1999b). Its sanctioning power includes the ability to revoke premarket approval, recall or seize products, and initiate criminal prosecutions (DHHS, FDA 1993).

The FDA's oversight of a growing range of products has resulted from statutory changes, judicial interpretations, and the FDA's discretionary authority. In the area of biologics, the agency has incorporated new categories into its regulatory framework through discretion and informal policymaking. Before the 1970s and 1980s, the FDA declined to regulate tissue and cellular material because it regarded this as part of the practice of medicine rather than as a biologic product. By the late 1980s, however, with HIV, hepatitis C, and other communicable diseases attracting public attention and with increasingly complex somatic cell gene therapies on the horizon, the CBER modified its policies (NBAC 1999b, 33–35). In 1984, it published a notice in the *Federal Register* asserting its authority over human gene therapies and stating it would subject gene therapies to the same regulations as other biologics (DHHS, FDA 1984). In this document, the agency invited researchers to contact the agency for earlier documents relating to "products of r-DNA technology." The agency reiterated it would continue its product-based approach; that is, it would assess r-DNA products the same way it assessed the safety and efficacy of other biologics.

The FDA issued more policy documents after 1984 that solidified its authority over somatic cell and gene therapies and provided further guidance about product development (Merrill and Javitt 2000). In 1991, it produced a guidance document listing points manufacturers and sponsors should consider in developing somatic cell and gene therapies (DHHS, FDA, CBER 1991). In 1993, it issued a policy statement defining somatic cell and gene therapy products as "analo-

TABLE 6.2 Therapies Regulated by the FDA

Somatic cell therapies
"Autologous,[a] allogeneic,[b] xenogeneic[c] cells that have been altered in biological characteristics ex vivo to be administered to humans and applicable to the prevention, treatment, cure, diagnosis, or mitigation of disease or injuries."

Gene therapies
"Products containing genetic material administered to modify or manipulate the expression of genetic material to alter the biological properties of living cells."[d]

[a] The patient's own cells are removed, modified, and injected.
[b] Human donor cells are modified and injected.
[c] Animal donor cells are modified and injected.
[d] The categories are not mutually exclusive. Products can be both somatic cell and gene therapies, such as somatic cells genetically altered outside the body and injected into the patient.

Source: U.S. Department of Health and Human Services, Food and Drug Administration, "Application of Current Statutory Authorities to Human Somatic Cell Therapy Products and Gene Therapy Products. Part II. Notice," *Federal Register* 58, no. 197 (14 October 1993): 53248.

gous products" that triggered review as drugs and/or biologics (DHHS, Public Health Service 1993). Reiterating its positions of 1984 and 1991, it defined somatic cell and gene therapies as depicted in Table 6.2. Around the same time that the FDA published its "Points to Consider" and other documents, the RAC was issuing its own "Points to Consider," as discussed in chapter 7.

The 1993 regulations required good manufacturing practices and careful record keeping to prevent the transmission of communicable diseases and to trace transmission if it occurred. In 1996, the CBER published an addendum to its 1991 "Points to Consider" document, focusing on the gene delivery system, and in 1998 it published a guidance document replacing the 1991 "Points to Consider" (DHHS, FDA, CBER 1998).

The FDA's oversight procedure begins formally when the manufacturer or investigator shifts from preclinical (nonhuman) research to clinical trials to test the product under development. Under the FDCA, drugs can be marketed for human use only if they are safe and efficacious for humans. Yet to prove safety and effectiveness, product testing on human subjects is necessary. Consequently, an exception in the law allows experiments to be conducted as long as human subjects are protected by regulations (Malinowski 2000, 216). To qualify for this exception, manufacturers or sponsors submit an IND. If, after reviewing the IND, FDA scientists are persuaded the product will likely be safe and effective when used with human subjects, the FDA will allow the study to proceed. Although the FDA's oversight officially begins with the IND submission, manufacturers are advised to consult earlier with the FDA. The *Food and Drug Administration Modernization Act* (FDAMA) of 1997 requires the FDA to work with investigators before the IND is submitted to work out problems and avoid delays (Food and Drug Law Institute 1998, 1; Malinowski 1999, 11.24). The IND process, which is the same for drugs and biologics, has evolved into a key part of FDA oversight.

The process of planning and submitting an IND, conducting tests after the investigator is allowed to proceed, and securing approval to market a drug can take years. The average time for a new drug to reach the market is fifteen years, and the effort can cost $500 million or more (T. Smith 1999, 139). By one estimate, it takes one to three years to get the necessary information together to submit an IND, two to ten years for clinical research on humans after investigators have been allowed to proceed, and two months to three years for review of the NDA (Zoon 1999).

The IND documents the scientific quality of the proposed clinical studies and the likelihood they will yield the needed data. It contains the investigator's commitment to submit protocols for institutional review board (IRB) oversight (21 C.F.R. 312.23 [a][iv]). Sponsors must show the research plan for the next year and the rationale, kinds of trials, expected risks, side effects, and summary of pharmacological and toxicological effects on animals, if any. Because agreements reached between investigators and authorities are binding, the FDA cannot impose heightened expectations later (Food and Drug Law Institute 1998, v).

Research to establish a drug's safety and efficacy proceeds through the following investigative, preclinical, and clinical stages (Fletcher 2000a):

Stage 1. Investigative (basic research)
Stage 2. Preclinical research using animals and human tissues
Stage 3. Clinical trials using human subjects
Phase I. Safe dosage levels (establish safety)
Phase II. Safety and effectiveness (establish efficacy)
Phase III. Large group studies (confirm efficacy)

In the investigative stage, researchers frame ideas, form hypotheses, and carry out basic research on cells or tissues without using animal or human subjects. In the preclinical stage, they test a product's likely safety and efficacy with animals, computer models, and/or human cells in laboratories. Preclinical research on animals exposes the animals to increasingly larger doses of the drug. Toxicity tests help determine whether it is safe to proceed to human subjects. Detailed regulations exist to guide researchers, protect human and animal subjects, and ensure high-quality research (Fletcher 2000a; T. Smith 1999, 140). In the clinical trials stage, researchers use human subjects to test the safety and effectiveness of the product.

The FDA will allow clinical trials to commence only if the IND shows that human subjects will be protected and that scientific evaluation is rigorous enough to allow the drug's effectiveness and safety to be evaluated. In reviewing the IND, FDA scientists look for procedures to protect human subjects, safety, scientific quality of the planned studies, and the likelihood the studies will yield enough information to enable a decision about marketing (21 C.F.R. 312.11). If the research is funded by the federal government, investigators must also follow the funding agency's own rules for protecting human subjects. If the research is not funded by the federal government, the oversight of the FDA, along with that of the sponsor's IRB, stands alone.

Clinical investigations using human subjects proceed in a three-step process. Phase I trials are designed to find the maximum safe dose of a new drug or biologic. Subjects at the beginning of Phase I trials receive doses of the drug well below those harmful to animals, and those at the middle and later stages receive higher doses until a maximum safe dose is established (T. Smith 1999, 142; Brody 1998, 169). The research is not intentionally therapeutic; human subjects are to be told they may not receive any benefit from the trial and may, in fact, experience adverse effects. Some volunteers are healthy; others have the disease the drug is developed to treat and want to take part in a study that holds hope for later therapy. During Phase I studies, investigators look for the action of the drug and side effects of different doses. They may look for signs of effectiveness, but Phase I studies are primarily geared to establishing safety and getting enough information to move to Phase II studies. Usually twenty to eighty subjects and patients are involved (21 C.F.R. 312.21). Approximately seventy percent of drugs in process fail at the Phase I stage (Malinowski 1999, 11.19).

Investigators in Phase II trials give a small number of research subjects (several hundred) who have the disease or condition the maximum tolerated safe dose of the drug to determine its effectiveness (T. Smith 1999, 143). Phase II studies determine whether the drug is safe for patients, and data from the studies are also used to determine the recommended dosages. These are double-blind ("placebo controlled") studies (21 C.F.R. 312.21 [b][2]).

Phase III trials involve a larger group of subjects—several hundred to several thousand, but usually around 1,000 to 2,000—to get a more statistically valid indicator of the drug's safety and effectiveness. These studies aim to obtain more information about effectiveness and safety so that the manufacturer can evaluate benefits and risks and label the drug accurately (21 C.F.R. 312.21 [2][c]). These studies generally compare the new drug with existing drugs. One group of subjects receives the new drug, a second group receives an existing drug or treatment, and a third group receives a placebo. The studies are ideally double blinded, so neither the participants nor the administering physicians know what group the subjects are in. Phase III trials take an average of four years and are often organized by pharmaceutical companies in centers within or across nations (T. Smith 1999, 144). Subjects in Phase II and III experiments may benefit from the research if they fall into the experimental rather than the control group.

After being satisfied that Phase III trials demonstrate the drug's safety and efficacy, the manufacturer submits an NDA or its equivalent if it is a biologic (biologics license application [BLA]) to CBER. An NDA or BLA is a detailed report containing all the information the manufacturer knows about the product. The BLA and NDA have the same bottom line—to show the product is "safe and effective for its labeled indication" (Malinowski 1999, 11.23). The agency must either approve the application or give notice for a hearing on a proposed denial within 180 days. The 180-day period starts when the FDA concludes it contains sufficient information. This adds sixty days to determine whether the application has been filed, so it is really 248 days. There are other exceptions too, which means the 180-day rule is not absolute (Malinowski 1999, 11.25). If the FDA gives premarket approval, the drug goes into production, with labeling and instructions. Phase IV studies may or may not be conducted after marketing to evaluate the drug's effectiveness, side effects, advantages, adverse effects, and reasons some patients do not respond.

If clinical studies do not meet the criteria for safety and efficacy, the FDA can place a clinical hold on the study or suspend an ongoing study. It can do this if the study exposes participants to an "unreasonable and significant risk of illness or injury," uses investigators who are not qualified, or uses a misleading brochure (21 C.F.R. 312.42). In 1997, for example, the FDA placed a preemptive clinical hold on all studies using pig cells and tissues on human subjects after receiving reports that retroviruses in the pig could infect human cells in vitro. The sponsors were told to develop ways to detect the viruses before proceeding (DHHS, FDA, CBER 1998, 15).

In 1996, the agency placed a clinical hold on an ongoing gene therapy study using female subjects when concerns arose that the genetic intervention might affect the oocytes of the women and be passed to the participants' later offspring. During the hold, researchers conducted studies with mice and found that a parallel intervention did not affect the germ cells of the male or female mice, and the clinical hold was lifted (Ye et al. 1998). In 2000, the FDA suspended seven ongoing trials at the University of Pennsylvania using gene therapy with adenovirus as a vector after a research participant, Jesse Gelsinger, died in a Phase I study conducted at the university's Institute for Human Gene Therapy (Marshall 2000a, 565).

Investigators who proceed with a study for which an IND has not been approved are subject to criminal or civil sanctions. The secretary of the DHHS under the Clinton administration, Donna Shalala, advocated legislation to authorize the FDA to impose monetary fines of up to $250,000 per investigator and up to $1 million per institution for violating informed consent and other research provisions (Shalala 2000, 810).

REPRODUCTIVE AND THERAPEUTIC SOMATIC CELL NUCLEAR TRANSFER

The FDA's highly structured regulatory code contrasts to the political complexities in Congress regarding therapeutic SCNT and ES cell research. When the idea of FDA oversight arose during debates over reproductive and therapeutic SCNT, it was greeted with relief by some and skepticism by others. After Richard Seed announced his intention to bring together scientists to clone a human, on January 8, 1998, President Clinton's press secretary, Mike McCurry, reassured worried policymakers that the FDA's authority to regulate gene and cell therapies extended to reproductive cloning. During the same press conference, DHHS Secretary Donna Shalala said that the FDA's role in protecting public safety and health meant "no one could go forward [with cloning] without submitting a request to the FDA." Later, two days before the scheduled cloture vote in the Senate, the FDA's deputy commissioner for external affairs, Sharon Smith Holston, sent a letter to Sen. Edward M. Kennedy asserting the FDA's authority to oversee clinical studies using cloning technology (Smith Holston 1998).

Smith Holston wrote that clinical research could proceed only if an IND were in effect and that the FDA would allow an IND to proceed only if the sponsor demonstrated safety and effectiveness through nonclinical research and showed a plan for conducting clinical research. Because cloning's safety and efficacy remained primitive and had not been established in animals, an IND would not likely be allowed to proceed. This would put a brake on contemplated clinical trials. In addition, by law, a sponsor would have to wait at least thirty days after submitting an IND to proceed, wrote Holston.

The FDA reasserted its authority over SCNT later in the year after the agency learned of studies in which investigators would transfer the nuclei of egg cells to enucleated eggs to help older women conceive. This was not cloning, but it would involve nuclear transfer. The premise of the studies was that characteristics of the cytoplasm of older women's eggs contributed to the difficulty older women have in conceiving. If the nucleus from an older woman's egg could be transferred to the enucleated egg of a younger woman, the newly composed egg could enable her to bear her genetically related child (Kolata 1997b). Hearing of these planned studies, Stuart L. Nightingale, the FDA's associate commissioner for health affairs, sent letters to chairs of IRBs across the country asserting the agency's authority over "clinical research using cloning technology to create a human being" (Nightingale 1998). Nightingale reminded investigators they must submit an IND to the FDA before proceeding with clinical studies using "cloning technology." Although the letter did not define cloning technology, the term appeared to encompass the transfer of any human somatic cell nucleus to an enucleated egg.

The FDA asserted its authority again in 1999, when Philip Noguchi, director of CBER's Division of Cellular and Gene Therapies, testified before and submitted a memorandum to the NBAC as it deliberated on ES cell issues (Noguchi 1999). Noguchi said the products over which the FDA had authority were broad enough to cover human clinical studies involving human cloning and human ES cells: "The definitions for somatic cell and gene therapies are sufficient to cover not only 'conventional' cell and gene therapy, but also human cloning and human embryonic pluripotent stem cells." Thus, the FDA used its discretionary judgment broadly to interpret somatic cell and gene therapies to include reproductive SCNT, therapeutic SCNT, ES cell therapies, and other forms of nuclear transfer. A cell that was subject to more than minimal manipulation and created to cure or treat a disease or condition was a biologic and subject to the expectations related to an IND. Congress had added the "or condition" part to the FDAMA in 1997 "with little debate or discussion." If reproductive SCNT could be said to circumvent the "condition" of infertility, this arguably would enable regulation of the practice (NBAC 1999b, 33).

The FDA has also situated itself for oversight of beginning-of-life technologies through its unified framework for regulating human cellular- and tissue-based products. Historically, conducting product oversight through a "patchwork of regulatory policies," CBER developed in the 1990s a "single regulatory program" to regulate human cellular- and tissue-based products in order to prevent the spread of infectious diseases (DHHS, FDA 1997). The program relies on a tiered-risk approach. Assuming that products pose differing risks of communicating disease, the approach stipulated that the greater the risk, the greater the regulation. Tissues and cells that are more than minimally manipulated and pose a higher risk are more extensively regulated than those with lesser manipulation and posing a lower risk. Products that are less risky traditionally do not need premarket approval, although they must meet minimum standards for infectious disease testing and processing. All other cellular- and tissue-based products must go through the traditional premarket approval process.

The first part of the comprehensive approach, proposed on May 14, 1998, and made final on January 19, 2001, creates a unified system for the registration of human cellular- and tissue-based products (human cell products) (DHHS, FDA 2001b). It requires manufacturers of human cell products to register with CBER so that a database of the names, addresses, and products of the manufacturers can be set up. Manufacturers are defined as "persons who recover, screen, test, process, store, label, package, or distribute" human cell products. The database is designed to enable officials to develop the tiered-risk method, send information about policies and risks to manufacturers, and conduct inspections.

The second part of the approach, announced September 30, 1999, would require most donors of cell products intended for transfer or transplantation to be tested for communicable diseases (DHHS, FDA 1999). The third part, announced January 8, 2001, would require manufacturers of human cell products to follow current good tissue practice (CGTP), which covers "proper handling, processing, storage, and labeling of human cellular and tissue-based products, record keeping, and the establishment of a quality program" (DHHS, FDA 2001a).

Of significance in this discussion of reproductive SCNT is the door the comprehensive approach opens for FDA oversight of reproductive products in the United States. Heretofore, the agency had regarded interventions in fertility clinics as part of the practice of medicine. Because the FDA regulated the development of products rather than medical practice, this created a hands-off orientation (NBAC 1999b, 35). The comprehensive approach, however, defined human cellular and tissue-based products as "medical products derived from the human body and used for replacement, *reproductive*, or therapeutic purpose" (DHHS, FDA 1998, 1–2; emphasis added).

With the second part of the approach, the FDA brought spermatozoa, eggs, and embryos for the first time under its purview, albeit in a limited manner. It supposed that infectious disease can spread by donating, processing, and storing reproductive cells and tissues. If cells are more than minimally manipulated, combined with nontissues, used for other than the usual purpose, or used for metabolic processes, they will be products subject to IND requirements (NBAC 1999a, 95).

The third part of the approach, released for public comment in January 2001, made the coverage of reproductive cells and tissues more explicit (DHHS, FDA 2001a). It required that CGTP would apply to sperm banks and ART facilities, which it defined as infertility clinics and andrology and embryology laboratories. It counted 330 ART facilities and 110 sperm banks in the country and it showed that 80 percent of ART facilities already conformed with CGTPs as a result of standards in the industry, accreditation programs, state licensing, and ASRM guidelines. It reported that 20 percent of the sperm banks already complied, and this 20 percent accounted for 95 percent "of all production." The FDA argued that shoddy practices in fertility facilities might contribute to low pregnancy and birth rates and let it be known it wanted stricter standards in the "reproductive tissue industry." Aiming for better quality assurance, it proposed greater agency involvement in the manipulation and transfer of reproductive cells and tissues. The standards allow discretion of producers by the use of flexible language, such as "suitable" and "appropriate" (ASRM 2001).

THE FOOD AND DRUG ADMINISTRATION'S ROLE IN CLONING POLICY

The FDA plays a narrowly crafted role in cloning policy. Its role is circumscribed by law; FDA oversight only comes into play when investigators intend to introduce a product to the market that fits into a category established by statute, is related to interstate commerce, and involves clinical trials using human subjects. The oversight procedure, set forth in the *Code of Federal Regulations*, revolves around documents in which investigators demonstrate that the products are safe and effective for clinical research (IND) or the marketplace (NDA or BLA). When research or marketing is allowed to proceed, safety and effectiveness are not guaranteed, but the preparatory research is designed to ensure that as much as possible is done to protect citizens from unsafe and ineffective biologics, drugs, and devices. Although the process is limited by law, the courts have broadly interpreted interstate commerce, and the FDA has broadly defined biologics and drugs. The agency has asserted that it has the authority to require the same approval process based on INDs for reproductive SCNT as for any other biologic. It has also reiterated that it will not allow reproductive SCNT to take place with questions of safety left unanswered.

The FDA's role is consistent with the United States as a market economy because the FDA is oriented to making products available as long as health protections are in place (U.S. Senate, CLHS-SPHS 1997c, 2). This leads to an ironic situation, however, because FDA involvement in reproductive SCNT is predicated for regulatory purposes on the notion that the human embryo is a more-than-minimally-manipulated cellular product. Given the intense division in the country regarding the moral status of the embryo—what John Fletcher calls the "dichotomous moral spheres within one country"— this odd outcome suggests that FDA involvement fits into only part of the policy picture (Fletcher 2000a, E6).

Still, in several ways FDA involvement is appropriate for developments in reproductive SCNT and related techniques. For one thing, it provides a framework that can be used for an array of innovative technologies. In contrast to efforts in Congress to target a single technology such as SCNT, the FDA's apparatus allows it to review a variety of products over time. The agency's oversight is proactive because it anticipates a group of related technologies and issues rules and guidance documents for managing innovation. FDA policy statements are separate from the daily administration of the IND/NDA process.

The incremental nature of FDA policy conforms with the incremental nature of scientific research. Administrative oversight is consistent with scientific inquiry because the officials who develop guidance documents and read and evaluate INDs are scientists themselves. The requirements for double-blind, placebo-based studies reflect high standards of scientific research. The agency can shut down programs, rescind an IND, or impose sanctions on research programs that do not meet these standards. It can also put manufacturers on notice that some biologics will not likely result in IND approval.

The incremental nature of FDA policymaking is, in its own way, open to public view and comment. Typically, the CBER will develop procedures and policies, publish them in the *Federal Register*, solicit public comments for ninety days, and issue final rules or actions after considering public comments. The agency also publishes nonbinding guidance documents that investigators usually follow as practical guides for novel research and that "become dogma in the field of biotechnology" (DHHS, FDA, RAC 1999; Carter 1996, 2376). These documents are available to all researchers through the Internet (www.fda.gov/cber/publications.htm) and other places.

The FDA acts under two sources of power: enabling statutes that establish its legitimacy and expectations that the FDA will, as an administrative agency, exercise discretion in interpreting these statutes (Fox 1997, 6). Courts have generally deferred to FDA discretion, with a notable exception being the U.S. Supreme Court's ruling that the FDA had exceeded its authority under the FDCA when it said it could regulate tobacco (*Food and Drug Administration et al. v. Brown & Williamson Corp. et al.* 529 US 120 [2000]). The agency used its discretionary power to monitor innovative somatic cell and gene therapy products in the early 1990s and it elected not to regulate ARTs in the 1980s and 1990s (NBAC 1999b, 31). It also used its discretion to assert that nuclear transfer technologies would fall under its purview. Expanding and contracting authority can be done expeditiously in that it is easier to change guidance documents than to change the law (Carter 1996, 377). In the case of the nuclear transfer, the initial assertion took the form of a letter sent to IRB chairs throughout the country.

A merit of FDA oversight comes from its parallels with administrative mechanisms in other countries. With international research collaborations more frequent, administrative procedures provide a common regulatory base for investigators. For example, efforts are underway in the European Union to provide consistent oversight of biotechnologies and to bring a harmonization of regulations. The European Medicines Evaluation Agency, the European equivalent of the FDA, establishes criteria for regulation through European Directives (EDs) (Malinowski 1999, 11.46). The EDs provide the basis for national laws; when the laws of all member states are consistent with the EDs, the standards are "harmonized." Drugs approved by the European Medicines Evaluation Agency are then accepted by all member states.

It has been observed that U.S. investigators must produce more documentation to proceed to Phase II clinical trials than investigators in Europe and, for this reason, many U.S. biotechnology companies conduct their Phase I clinical trials in Europe (Malinowski 1999, 10.44). A 1995 study showed that nearly three-quarters of the drugs approved by the FDA had already been approved in other countries (p. 10.44). For those who see documentation requirements as an indicator of human subjects' protection, the FDA's standards are advantageous. For those who see it as an unnecessary brake on development, the standards are a disadvantage. In either case, the common language of administration arguably provides a method of international collaboration to bridge disparities among national laws relating to reproductive SCNT and related technologies. FDA oversight extends to privately funded researchers and, in so doing, fills a policy need. In the case of reproductive or therapeutic SCNT, where federal money will not be forthcoming, and ES cell research where federal money is unlikely to be abundant, the FDA is the sole national overseer. Where national legislation is absent, elusive, or in process, administrative law allows oversight for safety and effectiveness of human cell products.

One drawback to FDA oversight is the unsettled question of whether the FDA has statutory authority to oversee reproductive SCNT. For one thing, it is arguable whether an embryo created through SCNT is a biologic product when an embryo created through IVF is not. If the FDA treats embryos differently because of the process through which they were created, this contravenes the agency's tradition of examining products for safety and efficacy regardless of the process by which they were created. As it said when asserting its authority over products of r-DNA in 1984, "[r]egulations by FDA must be based on the rational and scientific evaluation of products, and not on *a priori* assumptions about certain processes" (DHHS, FDA 1984, 50880). One FDA response is that an embryo created through SCNT meets its criteria for a product because it is more than minimally manipulated and has a systemic purpose other than that for which it was created.

It is also questionable whether reproductive SCNT treats, cures, or prevents a "condition." While infertility may well be a condition, individuals may use reproductive SCNT for reasons other than infertility. And even if the individual were infertile, reproductive SCNT would circumvent that condition but would not treat, cure, or prevent it. Moreover, the very flexibility that enables quick FDA oversight may also reflect loose adherence to definitions and concepts. The letter sent by Nightingale to IRB chairs seemed to equate nuclear transfer with cloning, when the technology in question related to the transfer of an egg nucleus to an enucleated egg. The statutory basis for asserting authority over egg cell nuclear transfer was not explained in that letter or subsequently. Until or unless the FDA's authority is contested in court, the scope of its authority remains unclear. A possible remedy is to make FDA oversight legally explicit by, for example, amending the FDCA (see, e.g., U.S. House 2001b).

In addition, while FDA oversight extends to privately funded projects, and thereby fills a gap in national policy, it nevertheless extends only where investigators intend to develop a product to treat a human disease or condition and use clinical trials to develop that product. Oversight presumably would not cover investigations before clinical trials or activities of practitioners in private infertility clinics who have no intention of marketing a product (NBAC 1999a, 93). This means an ad hoc study, in which a technician creates an embryo through SCNT and transfers it to a woman's uterus, is not covered if a clinic calls reproductive SCNT an innovative practice rather than research or product development (S. Cohen 1997, 28). Still, the question is open for discussion. In July 2001, the FDA sent a letter to selected researchers warning that the use of "genetically modified cells" secured through nuclear transfer, ooplasm transfer, or other listed means would be a clinical investigation requiring an IND. The letter seemed to indicate that any ad hoc use would be covered (Zoon 2001).

A third difficulty is that although FDA administrators review consent processes designed to protect the autonomy of research participants, the FDA's "ethics blind" enabling statutes caution agency scientists not to make ethical judgments on how products are used (NBAC 1999b, 31). To Rep. Billy Tauzin (R-LA) and others, this underscores the insufficiency of FDA oversight. If and when reproductive SCNT is regarded as safe, Tauzin argues, the FDA loses its potency as a brake. As Tauzin puts it, "I would not want to rely upon the single reed of Federal regulation to address experiments intended to create a baby from cloning technology" (U.S. House, Committee on Energy and Commerce, Subcommittee on Oversight and Investigations 2001, 5).

A fourth difficulty of relying on the FDA is the agency's legal obligation to respect trade secrets, which means agency oversight of early product development takes place within a zone of secrecy. Protecting the proprietary interests of manufacturers became a public issue when, after the death of Jesse Gelsinger in a gene therapy trial, the FDA faced criticism for not revealing adverse events from previous gene therapy trials. Although it subsequently proposed reforms to make information available on preclinical toxicity, adverse events, and previous FDA investigations in gene therapy trials, secrecy still prevails to preserve manufacturers' economic incentives to develop products (Kaiser 2001, 572).

CONCLUSIONS

FDA involvement is a key part of the existing regulatory apparatus. Those inclined to use existing resources as an alternative to restrictive legislation would see FDA oversight as an established and efficient system that meets basic safety and public health needs. According to this perspective, a product-based evaluation is especially appropriate where harms of an as yet unpracticed technique are speculative and difficult to quantify. Those inclined to a more active governmental role would see FDA involvement as removed from broader societal concerns that are at the heart of problematic technologies.

The merits of FDA oversight include its capacity to provide a conceptual umbrella for categories of innovative techniques, its science-based oversight, its tie to statutes enacted by Congress, and its ability to reach privately sponsored clinical trials involving reproductive and therapeutic SCNT. Its drawbacks include its link with product development, which casts a technical gaze over issues with significant normative features; questions about its statutory authority over reproductive SCNT; and the limited transparency for product development. In either case, the FDA engages in an often unheralded form of oversight that reminds us that legislation is only one method of monitoring reproductive SCNT and other innovative technologies. To say there is no cloning policy in the United States is to overlook the detailed FDA regulatory structure that has already been activated.

CHAPTER 7

OVERSIGHT THROUGH FEDERAL RESEARCH FUNDING

The policy apparatus related to the federal funding of research using human participants (clinical trials) contributes to the normative and procedural backdrop of a cloning policy. Because the federal government does not fund reproductive or therapeutic SCNT, the apparatus operates in the shadows. It is, however, activated if privately funded researchers voluntarily respect federal guidelines, or it could be activated if Congress were to require all clinical researchers, regardless of funding source, to follow federal guidelines. Even if neither of these happens, the apparatus contributes to expectations about the ethical conduct of inquiry into innovative reproductive and genetic technologies.

NATURE OF FEDERAL PROTECTION OF HUMAN RESEARCH PARTICIPANTS

Vigorous protections for human research participants are rooted in the Nuremberg Code of 1947, which was framed in response to Nazi human rights violations during World War II. Central to the code is the principle that participation in research must be voluntary ("Nuremberg Code" 1995). The Declaration of Helsinki, adopted by the World Medical Association in Helsinki in 1964 and revised in Tokyo in 1975 and Venice in 1983, reinforced the principles of the Nuremberg Code and added to the requirements for informed consent ("Declaration of Helsinki" 1995). In the United States, after it was revealed that informed consent had been violated in various studies, including most patently the Tuskegee syphilis study, Congress passed the *National Research Act of 1974*. This law set up a system to review all research protocols funded by the DHEW and involving human subjects.

The apparatus has as its core IRBs set up at the institutions of investigators and made up of at least five members, including at least one scientist, one nonscientist, and one person from outside the research institution. The IRB system places initial authority in the institution, where the members are presumed to be familiar with local professional standards and priorities of the institution (45 C.F.R. 46.107). IRBs examine protocols, consent forms, and other materials to ensure that the clinical investigation complies with federal standards to protect research participants. After the IRB signs off, the protocol moves to the institution's administration and then to the funding agency where it is reviewed by peers and agency administrators. At least once a year, IRBs review protocols and reports prepared by investigators, and they look for harms to participants (adverse events) and unexpected problems (45 C.F.R 46.109e; 21 C.F.R. 56.1092). Policymakers periodically refine IRB regulations in response to problems and changing conditions (see, e.g., Cohen 2000).

The *National Research Act of 1974* also created the National Commission for the Protection of Human Subjects of Biomedical and Behavioral Research to examine policies relating to research subjects, recommend improvements, and identify the basic ethical principles that underlie all human biomedical research. After extensive meetings, the commission drafted its report at the Belmont Center outside Baltimore. This report, released in 1979 and known as the Belmont Report, identified ethical principles to govern research using human subjects (National Commission for the Protection of Human Subjects of Biomedical and Behavioral Research 1995). Beneficence directs researchers to maximize benefits and minimize harms; justice requires a fair distribution of the benefits and risks of research; and respect for persons recognizes the dignity and autonomy of individuals and requires informed consent to participate in research studies. The resulting guidelines aimed to protect subjects and guide research (Williams 1996, 174).

Of the federal departments that fund research on human subjects, the DHHS is the primary source of funding for biomedical research, and the NIH is the most active biomedical funding agency within the DHHS. Located in Bethesda, Maryland, the NIH contains twenty-four funding institutes that receive independent appropriations, including the National Cancer Institute, National Institute on Aging, National Institute of Mental Health, and National Eye Institute. The most recent addition is the National Institute of Biomedical Imaging and Bioengineering, signed into law in late 2000. The NIH supports research conducted intramurally by scientists employed at the NIH, and extramurally by researchers at universities, research facilities, and other institutions. The NIH is the single largest source of biomedical research funds in the United States. Over one-half the funds allocated for research in the country go to biomedical investigations (Malakoff 1999).

The year after the National Commission issued its first biennial report in 1981, the Office of Science and Technology Policy proposed that all federal departments and agencies should adopt a common core of regulations governing human subjects research based on DHHS rules (DHHS et al. 1991, 28004; McCarthy 1995, 2289). This would make uniform the federal regulations that had varied among the agencies and departments. A proposed model federal policy for protection of human subjects was published in the *Federal Register* for public comment in 1986. A revised model appeared in 1988, and the final version appeared in 1991, codified as 45 C.F.R. 46. Seventeen agencies and departments have agreed to adopt what came to be known as the Common Rule. Agreement obligates each agency and department to bring its own regulations into conformity with the Common Rule. The FDA published parallel rules in 1981 and 1988 at the same time as did DHHS, and it issued its own final rule at the same time as the Common Rule, codified as 21 C.F.R. 50 and 56. The FDA conforms to the Common Rule but, because it and the other agencies have different missions, has not officially adopted it (NIH 1999a).

The Common Rule applies if three criteria are met. First, the investigation must be "research," which is defined in the regulations as a "systematic investigation including development, testing, and evaluation designed to develop or contribute to generalizable knowledge" (45 C.F.R. 46.102[d]). An ad hoc inquiry or an experimental treatment is not generally regarded as research. Second, the research must take place in an institution that has signed an "assurance" with the government. An assurance obligates an institution to comply with the federal rules for protecting participants in research. An assurance signed for one grant is a single project assurance; when signed for multiple grants, it is a multiple grant assurance. With a multiple assurance, institutions promise that all their researchers will abide by regulations even if the projects are funded privately. Over 4,000 universities, hospitals, and research institutions in the United States had negotiated assurances with the NIH's Office of Protection from Research Risks (OPRR) as of 1999 (DHHS 1999, 1). The FDA's equivalent of the Common Rule differs here because it covers all clinical studies leading to product development, including those funded by private sources.

Third, human subjects must be involved, defined in the regulations as "living individual[s]" about whom the researcher will obtain data through an intervention or interaction or from "identifiable private information" (45 C.F.R. 46.102[f][2]). Persons at IVF clinics who donate embryos, sperm, or eggs for research that can be traced to them, thereby making them identifiable, are research subjects. These persons would be research subjects if an intervention were performed on them in the process of research. Embryos are not human subjects, however, because they are not living individuals under the law.

Until 2000, the OPRR oversaw the regulatory apparatus for research involving humans and animals. Among other things, it negotiated assurances with research institutions and ensured that the institutions set up IRBs to review all human subjects research regardless of the funding source. The OPRR investigated compliance with procedures and had the authority to suspend all federally funded human subjects research at institutions not following federal guidelines (NIH 1999b, 2). In the late 1990s, the OPRR was unusually active and shut down clinical research programs at a number of highly respected medical centers (Spicer 2000, 262). It also started a comprehensive review of gene therapy protocols at the University of Pennsylvania in response to a participant's death in a gene therapy trial (Marshall 2000a, 566). In 2001, the OPRR's successor, the Office for Human Research Protections, shut down all clinical trials at Johns Hopkins University School of Medicine after a participant in a Phase I asthma trial died as an apparent result of inhaling a drug used in the study (Kolata 2001).

Amid concerns that federal regulations to protect research subjects ought to be strengthened, OPRR set up a review panel to examine the issues and make recommendations. In 1999, the OPRR Review Panel issued a report recommending that the OPRR be moved from the NIH, where it had been located since 1972, to the DHHS. The move was aimed at heightening the office's stature, improving its leadership potential for the seventeen agencies that adhere to the Common Rule, and giving it more opportunities to initiate policy. In addition, the move was designed to avoid the perception that the OPRR, as an agency of the NIH, was biased in favor of the research process (Marshall 1999, 1751). In June 2000, the office was moved to the Office of Public Health and Science in the office of the secretary of DHHS and renamed the Office for Human Research Protections (OHRP).

The DHHS secretary announced a series of other initiatives in May 2000 to improve protection mechanisms for research partici-pants. These initiatives related to education and training of clinical investigators and IRB members, improvement of informed consent procedures, greater monitoring of Phase I and Phase II clinical trials, clarification of conflict of interest standards, and consideration of proposals to fortify the FDA's sanctions (Shalala 2000; Spicer 2000). The DHHS also formed a twelve-person National Human Research Protections Advisory Committee to advise the DHHS secretary.

HEIGHTENED OVERSIGHT FOR CATEGORIES OF RESEARCH

When biomedical research poses especially complex issues of safety and ethics, the government may impose heightened oversight of clin-ical research, which takes the form of an additional layer of review by a body set up explicitly for this purpose. The review also includes dis-cussion of ethical as well as scientific issues. As discussed below, the government successfully initiated an added layer of review for gene therapy via the RAC. It unsuccessfully attempted to add a layer of review for human embryo research via the EAB. Efforts to add extra review for ES cell studies are still in process.

Gene Therapy and the Recombinant DNA Advisory Committee

Scientists' refinement in 1973 of the procedures for recombining DNA in organisms led to concerns that genetically modified organisms could inadvertently infiltrate into the environment. Concerned about inadvertent release, scientists convened a meeting at the Asilomar Center in California to discuss ways of containing organisms while the risks were assessed. At the Asilomar meeting, participants crafted a four-part containment model designed to impose graduated restrictions according to the risks posed by recombinant DNA (r-DNA) research. They also recommended that the NIH set up a special research oversight committee to develop guidelines and review research proposals to ensure that hazardous organisms were not mistakenly released. The government endorsed the proposal and established the RAC in 1974. As requested, the RAC developed guidelines, completed in 1976, to prevent the unintended release of genetically modified organisms. Investigators at institutions with government assurances were obligated to comply with the guidelines. Failure to do so would lead to the loss of federal funds.

The twenty-five-member RAC held public meetings, reviewed research proposals, and provided a forum for evaluating the risks of genetically modified organisms. The RAC's oversight complemented that of institutional biosafety committees (IBCs), which were set up at institutions where researchers received federal funding. Researchers seeking government funds submitted their proposals to the IBCs for their approval before sending the proposals to the RAC, granting agency, and other overseers for review. Although only those investigators seeking federal funds were obligated to submit proposals to IBCs and the RAC, the respect accorded containment regulations induced privately funded researchers voluntarily to submit proposals.

By the mid-1980s, scientists were moving toward their goal of using r-DNA technology on humans to treat disease. The prospects of modifying the genes of human cells for therapy provoked both excitement and safety concerns. Among other things, observers were wary about whether gene therapy would set the stage for future interventions on the human germ line. In response to these uncertainties, the RAC set up a working group to consider guidelines for human gene therapies. This led to the to the publication of questions for researchers to address before proceeding with clinical trials on gene therapy. The RAC's "Points to Consider in the Design and Submission of Human Somatic-Cell Gene Therapy Protocols" related to somatic cell gene therapy only; Appendix M stipulated that the NIH would not at that time entertain protocols for germ-line (inheritable) gene therapy (NIH 1985).

Early somatic cell gene therapy protocols involved efforts to add or replace genes to cells to replace a defective gene. In these studies, researchers identified and isolated the defective gene and then produced large quantities of a normal gene. They incorporated the normal gene into a delivery system or vector such as viruses modified not to produce a disease or to replicate themselves. When weakened, viruses, such as the cold virus (adenovirus), acted like vectors, described by one science writer as "taxicabs that drive healthy DNA into cells" (Stolberg 1999b, 137). Gene therapy researchers have had persistent problems getting enough genes into cells to make a difference; circumventing the body's defense system, which shuts down the genes once they enter the cells; getting genes into the right place in the cells; and making sure the correct amount of the protein is produced to treat the disease (Stolberg 1999a). For gene therapy to succeed, the synthetic genes must take over the programming of the protein.

The first proposed clinical trials involving gene therapy were marker studies that traced the path of the vector delivering the manipulated cells. Two studies were approved after undergoing some fifteen layers of review, including IRB review (human subjects were involved) and IBC review (r-DNA activities were involved). After IRB and IBC approval, the researchers submitted protocols to the granting agency, usually the NIH, for peer review and RAC review of projects involving the transfer of genetically engineered cells to human subjects. The Office of Recombinant DNA Activities was in charge of compliance.

The RAC provided a procedural mechanism to slow the research and development process and to oversee medical innovations raising greater than ordinary concerns about safety and ethics. Some but not all observers expected that heightened review would be phased out when safety concerns were met. The RAC periodically modified Appendix M to change the documentation investigators needed to submit and the questions they needed to address (Beach 1999, 51). The RAC had jurisdiction only over publicly funded research, but over one hundred corporations without federal funding voluntarily complied with the guidelines and some of them participated in RAC's open quarterly meetings. The sanction for publicly funded researchers or institutions not complying with the regulations was a loss of funds for r-DNA research.

By the mid-1990s, numerous gene therapy protocols had been approved. The safety of gene therapy did not at that time appear to be a problem, although gene therapy's effectiveness had not been demonstrated. The NIH director called for the RAC's dissolution, saying detailed review of protocols unnecessarily delayed research and that the intention had always been to fade RAC's procedural oversight (Marshall 1996). Pharmaceutical companies said the RAC was redundant because the FDA also reviewed gene therapy protocols (Stolberg 1999b, 139). A move to disband the RAC provoked dissent from those who thought heightened oversight was still needed and who endorsed the RAC's public role as a forum for discussing ethical and other issues. In 1996, it was decided the RAC would be retained but with a different composition and mission.

Under the new policy, the RAC was reduced from twenty-five members to fifteen, and it no longer had the authority to approve or disapprove of individual gene therapy protocols, which now were reviewed by IRBs and the FDA. The RAC would, however, conduct a full review of individual proposals if the NIH director, three or more RAC members, or other federal agencies recommended it. The RAC still functioned as a place where investigators would register gene therapy trials and file reports of adverse events. The RAC would discuss protocols at a public meeting if the protocol involved something new, such as a new delivery system, targeted disease, or application (DHHS, FDA, RAC 1999). At its December 1999 meeting, for example, RAC members voted to initiate full review of a gene therapy protocol for patients with early Alzheimer's disease. The protocol involved a disease of interest to the public that had not been previously subject to gene therapy. The protocol also raised ethical concerns about the ability of early Alzheimer's patients to consent to the study. RAC members expressed their concerns in writing, and the investigators addressed these concerns in writing before the meeting.

While the RAC lost much of its oversight authority with its revised mission, it also gained a policy role when it was authorized to hold gene therapy policy conferences (GTPCs) to oversee scientific and ethical issues raised by gene therapy research. Each policy conference was to address an ethical or scientific issue raised by gene therapy research. The RAC held three GTPCs by the end of 1999. One, in January 1999, dealt with gene therapy for fetuses (prenatal gene transfer). W. French Anderson and Esmail D. Zanjani submitted two "pre-proposals" for in utero (fetal) gene therapy, primarily to promote discussion of germ-line issues. During the two-day public conference on in utero gene therapy, speakers addressed scientific and ethical issues, among them the possibility that modifications on the fetus would pass to the fetal germ line and be inherited by future generations. Later, the RAC issued a statement concluding there were insufficient data from preclinical studies to start in utero gene therapy clinical trials. The RAC also identified numerous issues to be addressed before clinical trials could start, including the matter of inadvertent germ-line transmission (Zanjani and Anderson 1999).

The RAC held another gene therapy policy conference in late 1999 on the use of adenovirus as a vector for gene therapy. The one-day conference was held in conjunction with a regularly scheduled two-day RAC meeting after Jesse Gelsinger's death in a Phase I clinical trial of adenovirus gene therapy. Seven cohorts of two to four subjects each received progressively stronger doses of the manipulated gene. Gelsinger, the last recipient, had a mild and controlled form of the targeted disease. Two days after the injection, he died. It was subsequently revealed that two monkeys had died in preclinical trials and that human participants in the clinical trials had suffered toxic reactions. Gelsinger had not been informed of the monkey deaths during the consent process (Smaglik 2000, 584).

An overflow crowd attended the December 1999 gene therapy policy conference and RAC meeting. Issues included the safety of adenovirus, communications between the RAC and FDA, and the reporting of adverse events. Particular attention went to the reporting of adverse events in gene therapy, defined as life-threatening events or those that result in death, hospitalization, or significant disability.

In anticipation of the RAC meeting, the RAC and NIH proposed in the *Federal Register* a change in reporting adverse events that would require more events to be reported and at an earlier time.

Although the multiple layers of oversight required for gene therapy clinical trials have diminished in number over time, gene therapy trials are scrutinized more carefully than any other therapy, with oversight by the IRB, IBC, FDA, and Office of Biotechnology Activities. This contrasts with other clinical trials requiring only IRB and FDA review. With gene therapy, the government in effect determined that all experiments using humans were research and thereby subject to research controls (T. Smith 1999, 37). Still, Gelsinger's death revealed that the oversight was not as rigorous as procedures required. Following the death, the NIH contacted all gene therapy researchers who were using adenoviral vectors and found there had been 691 serious adverse events, but only thirty-nine of these had been reported to the NIH (Wadman 2000).

By 1999, the government had reviewed 331 gene therapy protocols involving over four thousand patients (Stolberg 1999b, 138). Over time, gene therapy has come to involve more than adding or replacing genes. Most trials use patients with severe diseases who have not responded to conventional therapies. The investigators remain at Phase I and Phase II studies primarily in order to establish the safety of gene delivery systems, although evidence of clinical benefit had started to emerge by 2000 (BIO 1999, 2; Kolata 2000). The regulatory apparatus expanded and contracted, with rigorous oversight in the first half of the decade and relaxed oversight in the second half.

Embryo Research and Heightened Review

Ethics Advisory Board

A second example of heightened oversight relates to efforts that were not instituted. In the mid-1970s in response to concerns about IVF, Congress passed a law stipulating that research on IVF could be funded by the DHEW only if it were reviewed by its EAB: "No application or proposal involving human in vitro fertilization may be funded by the Department until the application or proposal has been reviewed by the Ethics Advisory Board and the Board has rendered advice as to its acceptability from an ethical standpoint" (45 C.F.R. 46.204[d][1]).

In 1977, an investigator from Vanderbilt University submitted a proposal to fertilize human eggs in vitro and study them for chromosomal abnormalities to assess the safety of IVF. The NIH approved the proposal for funding in October 1977. Enacting the provisions of 45 C.F.R. 46, the DHEW secretary set up the cross-disciplinary EAB made up of thirteen members and two consultants. The EAB members were asked to consult with ethicists and others, solicit public comment, explore the issues raised by IVF, and disseminate the results, which they did by meeting in eleven cities and gathering testimony and statements from citizens and organized interest groups. In its 1979 report, the EAB concluded that IVF was ethically acceptable for married couples and that research on human embryos was acceptable when the research was designed to establish IVF safety, the question would yield important scientific information, the method complied with federal laws governing research on human subjects, tissue donors gave informed consent, and the embryos were not kept alive for more than fourteen days after fertilization. Researchers were obligated to inform the public if IVF were shown to harm fetuses. The EAB concluded that the "human embryo is entitled to profound respect, but this respect does not necessarily encompass the full legal and moral rights attributed to persons" (DHEW, EAB 1979).

In the year following the report's publication, the DHEW received over 12,000 letters, of which only 2 percent supported IVF, mainly on the grounds it would help infertile couples (Bonnicksen 1989, 80). The rest opposed IVF, regarding it as inherently immoral and wrongly ignoring the rights of the embryo. Following the report's release in 1979, the research proposal was denied, though not with an explicit letter, and the DHEW secretary tabled the EAB recommendations. The next DHEW secretary, who came to office in 1980, disbanded the EAB, which meant no research on IVF could be funded without the requisite EAB to review the proposals. Although not a ban on embryo research, the absence of an EAB amounted to a moratorium on the federal funding of research in which embryos were injured or destroyed.

Following the EAB's disbanding, whoever conducted embryo research did so in IVF clinics using private funding, but there was little evidence that research was underway. Later, in 1987, researchers from Washington University submitted a proposal to the NIH to study nonviable fertilized and unfertilized human eggs to study how to improve the culture medium used for fertilization. This was the first proposal sent to the NIH since the proposal from Vanderbilt ten years earlier (Norman 1988, 406). Although officials at NIH proposed in the *Federal Register* the establishment of a new EAB and solicited public comments, no board was instituted.

Recommendations of the Human Embryo Research Panel

Another attempt to change the embryo research funding policy occurred during the transition from the presidency of George Bush to that of Bill Clinton. During that time Congress lifted the EAB requirement for IVF research in a "barely noticed" section of the *NIH Revitalization Act of 1993* (Gianelli 1994, 3). With this proviso, Congress intended for embryo research to proceed. According to the Senate report that accompanied the bill to the floor, "Section 492A will permit the funding of peer reviewed and approved research proposals involving assisted reproductive technologies including in vitro fertilization (IVF)." Similarly, the House report stated that "Subsection c nullifies the de facto moratorium currently in place on federal support for research on human in vitro fertilization" (quoted in NIH 1994, 14).

Without the EAB requirement, embryo research theoretically could be funded with local IRB review. Before opening the research for funding, however, the acting director of the NIH, acting cautiously, established the HERP to review issues raised by embryo research, solicit public comment, and make recommendations about the ethical acceptability of various kinds of embryo research.

Nineteen panelists in science, ethics, law, social science, public health, and public policy made up the HERP. They were asked to give advice about what categories of embryo research were ethically acceptable, ethically unacceptable, or warranted further review. The panel held six public meetings in 1994, solicited public comments from 200 organizations and the public, commissioned four papers, heard forty-six oral presentations at its meeting, and received 30,000 written comments.

In its 111-page report, the panelists regarded some forms of research as ethically acceptable, within limits (NIH 1994). The studies would need to be conducted by qualified persons, promise "significant scientific or clinical benefit," and have objectives that could not be accomplished with research using animals or human gametes. Moreover, the studies must keep the number of embryos to a minimum, allow donors to know the nature and purpose of the research, not involve buying or selling of embryos or gametes, ensure an equitable selection of donors, and keep the research period as short as possible (not beyond the fourteenth day after fertilization). The HERP regarded the generation of embryos for research as ethically acceptable, within limits, as well as the use of embryos donated by couples in IVF programs.

The HERP recommended a three-stage review process for embryo research protocols involving an IRB, standard NIH review, and ad hoc review by a board set up by the NIH (NIH 1994, 3). The majority of panelists thought that an extra layer of review was needed because no human embryo research had ever been funded in the United States, leaving "virtually no experience with reviewing what in many instances will be complex and controversial research" (NIH 1994, 85). Moreover, IRB review would not be sufficient because issues raised by embryo research are those "about which IRBs have no special expertise" and because the sporadic nature of IRB review does not provide consistent review and accumulated precedents about embryo research. In addition, the NIH study sections were not sufficient because the reviewers attended to technical questions and did not have expertise in ethics. Over time, this layer of review could be lifted and the normal review process reinstituted. The NIH would publish a summary of funded studies twice a year with a comment on problems, if any. This review would be published in the NIH "Guide to Grants and Contracts" and sent to IRBs to help ensure consistency of guidelines. If controversial research proposals were received, the NIH could create ad hoc panels to review the issues raised.

On December 2, 1994, the HERP released its report, and before the day's end, President Clinton issued an Executive Order rejecting the most controversial part—funding to create human embryos for research—and directing the NIH director not to allocate money for projects involving the creation of embryos for research. He left the rest untouched and did not mention embryo research using embryos donated from IVF programs. In the ongoing legislative session, appropriations bills for the next fiscal year had been delayed (Varmus

2000, 51). Opponents of embryo research added an amendment to the NIH appropriations bill barring funding for projects in which embryos were created or harmed. Similar riders were added to all subsequent NIH appropriations bills.

Human Embryonic Stem Cell Research

The next effort to implement funding for embryo research came with the ES cell discoveries of late 1998, which, as discussed in chapter 5, spurred a political imbroglio for the Bush administration. Once again, those who believed embryo research amounted to the immoral destruction of living persons and those who believed research using embryos could address the sufferings of individuals locked forces in a heated and protracted controversy, only this time the lines were less clear cut. Proposals by the NIH and NBAC and some members of Congress would allow ES cell funding with tight procedural controls and heightened oversight. For example, a bill introduced by Sen. William Frist would allow ES cell research for a five-year period on a limited number of stem cell lines within a strong oversight system. Among other things, he proposed placing scientific review of stem cell research in the Institute of Medicine and creating an independent presidential advisory panel to "monitor evolving bioethical issues" related to stem cell research. Transparency would be realized through the DHHS via an annual report to Congress on federal funding, number of cell lines created, results, amount of funding, and information on number of applications received and granted (*Washington Fax* 2001a).

As it turned out, President Bush limited funding to previously existing ES cell lines. On the one hand, this limitation greatly truncated the breadth of fundable research. On the other hand, however, it introduced only minimal new regulations (NIH, Office of the Director 2001a). The mission of the PCB, the newly formed council, was broad and related to the airing of perspectives on various biomedical topics. Owing to the events of September 11, 2001, the president delayed formally establishing the PCB until late 2001 (President, Executive Order 2001). The PCB lacked regulatory authority, so no additional regulatory oversight for ES cell research had been initiated by the end of 2001.

HUMAN RESEARCH PROTECTIONS AND
REPRODUCTIVE SOMATIC CELL NUCLEAR TRANSFER

Federal protections of research subjects coalesce into a detailed, respected, comprehensive, and flexible regulatory framework. This system of oversight, which occupies a large section of the *Code of Federal Regulations*, has been refined periodically since its origins nearly thirty years ago and is familiar to scientists (Williams 1996, 170). The number of institutions with assurances extends the breadth of Common Rule protections considerably. Although technically the Common Rule regulations extend only to research funded by institutions that have signed assurances with the government, some private institutions voluntarily sign assurances with the government. This voluntary adherence by some privately funded researchers and the adoption of the IRB model by other national governments attest to the system's legitimacy. Based on principles articulated in the Belmont Report, the apparatus provides a more explicit bioethical component to oversight than does the FDA's regulatory apparatus, although the FDA and NIH share a history based on similar ethical principles (Williams 1996, 170).

The Common Rule apparatus governing human subjects research contributes a procedural framework that can be reformed as times change and needs dictate. In recent years, a recognition of the need to boost protections has spurred various initiatives to buttress protections for research subjects, including establishing the NBAC, upgrading the OHRP, subjecting IRBs to tighter controls, and establishing new conflict of interest standards (Marshall 2000c; Shalala 2000).

Federal regulations provide a strong policy resource for a nation with a robust biomedical research program. The system is a shadow apparatus for reproductive SCNT, ES cell studies, and related innovative technologies because the federal government does not fund studies in which human embryos are damaged or destroyed. IVF, preimplantation genetic diagnosis, and other ARTs have developed without funding oversight.

Federal oversight of embryo research could be activated in two ways. First, the government could open for funding categories of research, such as ES cell research. If the government were to more broadly fund ES cell studies, this would introduce Common Rule protections for the adults who donate gametes or embryos and also to participants in ES cell clinical trials. Even if only a narrow window for the derivation and/or use of new ES cell lines were opened, this would broaden expectations about appropriate informed consent procedures and, ideally, encourage voluntary compliance from investigators engaged in more expansive research. This policy change would also enhance the quality of research over time because it would open studies to the highly competitive funding process of the NIH and other institutes. Within this system, research applications are first reviewed by initial review groups made up of scientists from outside the government who rate applications by their scientific and technical merit.

Extending federal funding would also bring research to the public purview and encourage a broader dissemination of findings than occurs with corporate sponsors who maintain secrecy until patents have been filed. The growing tendency of pharmaceutical companies to use organizations that contract with research facilities rather than to work directly with scientists in academic centers further removes research from public view (Malinowski 2000, 224–25).

A primary difficulty in implementing this approach is the active constituency of individuals who hold that embryo research is morally illicit and should not be underwritten by the government. This makes federal funding of research into innovative reproductive technologies politically contentious. In addition, even with funding, the current apparatus would come into play only when "research" is conducted using "human subjects" at institutions with signed assurances with the government. If ad hoc innovative therapies are regarded as the practice of medicine rather than research, they need not be subject to IRB review. Corporations, privately funded researchers, and private fertility clinics fall outside the regulatory net if they are not engaging in product development and not conducting research as narrowly defined.

A second way of activating the federal apparatus is to bring all human research, no matter what the funding source, under federal controls. In its 1997 cloning report, the NBAC wrote in dicta that this would be a "robust response to new and unanticipated technological innovations" (NBAC 1997a, 99; Marshall 1997). The NBAC returned to the idea in its 2001 report, *Ethical and Policy Issues in Research Involving Human Participants*, by recommending, among other things, that Congress enact a law making federal oversight "available to participants in both publicly and privately sponsored research" (NBAC 2001). To implement this, an independent national-level human research office would be established by law. Policymakers would identify research not subject to federal oversight and determine whether it should be controlled.

Other policymakers have also recommended dropping distinctions between private and public research. For example, in June 2000, Rep. Diana DeGette (D-CO) introduced a bill, the *Human Research Subject Protections Act of 2000*, to bring all human research studies under a single standard "independent of setting and funding source" (Marshall 2000b). The bill, H.R. 4605, would amend the PHSA so the Common Rule would apply to all human subjects research. It would also establish a federal office to oversee this (U.S. House 2000).

A merit of bringing human research under federal control is that it would address the ironic situation in which research about a matter of keen public interest, such as ES cell studies, is not in the public eye because it is funded privately. It would also provide a guide for IRBs as they address novel technologies (Moreno and Tanner 1999). On the other hand, this would be a dramatic departure from biomedical research traditions, and it would generate formidable political hurdles (NBAC 1997a, 100). Unless it took the form of a "single federal agency with a single reporting mechanism," it would create a new workload for agencies that are already overextended and it would add to an already complex regulatory framework (Snyderman and Holmes 2000, 595). Any proposal for a new agency would be at odds with an administration generally favoring less rather than more regulation.

A more modest variation of this plan would be to use an existing agency, the RAC, to review protocols of all researchers, privately or publicly funded, related to innovative reproductive and genetic technologies. Ira Carmen, a political scientist and former RAC member, proposed this for reproductive SCNT in 1997 (Carmen 1997, 758), and the approach could be expanded to cover other techniques. In recent years, numerous observers have recommended revitalizing the RAC or establishing a RAC-like body to review all research involving IGMs (Palmer and Cook-Deegan in press; Frankel and Chapman 2000; 2001; Parens and Juengst 2001). With this plan, the RAC would be moved outside of the NIH to make it independent of funding sources. The RAC, following its history with gene therapy, could encourage public discussion on IGMs and, if research commences, subject protocols to ethical and scientific review (Palmer and Cook-Deegan in press). Presumably, a similar plan could be initiated for research involving SCNT if attitudes moderated and if the activities were not banned by law.

CONCLUSIONS

The federal government has a highly structured system to protect research participants and, as the gene therapy history shows, it may heighten the scrutiny for research of particular salience or for research that poses unusual risks. The structure is triggered by federal funding, and, in the absence of funding, it has been activated narrowly for ES cell research and it has not been activated for SCNT, comprehensive human ES cell studies, or related technologies. Even if activated, the basic model has a limited impact because it covers only human subjects taking part in research, which is defined as the systematic acquisition of knowledge, not ad hoc inquiries. Still, this would make the protocols public, allow the research to be tracked, and set a foundation for other plans to heighten oversight, such as establishing a registry for reviewing comprehensive ES cell research.

Activation is not taking place, however, as Congress weighs bills to withhold funding for SCNT research or to ban it altogether. The more that research moves into the private sector or to other nations, the less useful is this apparatus in the crafting of policy governing future innovative reproductive technologies.

CHAPTER 8

STATE LEGISLATURES AND
STATE AND FEDERAL COURTS

Policymaking is an enterprise based on incremental adjustments. While the adjustment of oversight mechanisms may not be elegant, it is realistic in a system such as that of the United States, where the political structure minimizes centralized power and where numerous places exist to add to and amend policy. These include state legislatures, which can play a role in regulating reproductive SCNT, and the courts, which may play a role in reviewing anticloning laws. The courts may still be drawn into policymaking even if reproductive SCNT is not specifically barred. For one thing, the possibility of an eventual acceptance of cloning cannot be dismissed. For another, citizens may conceive through SCNT in another nation, return with their children, and eventually be drawn into custody or inheritance disputes that require judicial intervention to resolve.

REPRODUCTIVE SOMATIC CELL NUCLEAR TRANSFER AND EMBRYO RESEARCH LAWS

In general, state laws that limit reproductive SCNT fall into three categories: new laws that specifically target reproductive cloning, laws that restrict embryo research, and laws related to the practice of ARTs. Of most immediate relevance are laws passed since 1997 that target reproductive cloning.

By early 1998, over half of the states had introduced bills to restrict reproductive cloning. These bills varied widely in their purpose, definition, substance, and method of enforcement (Greely 1998, 131). While most did not pass, six states by 2001 had enacted laws to limit human reproductive cloning. California was the first, in 1997 (Cal. Health & Safety Code sections 24185, 24187). Under its law, a medical practitioner who clones a human being risks losing his or her business license. A corporation or other facility engaged in reproductive cloning could be fined $1 million, and an individual could be fined $250,000. This law is both more and less restrictive than other bills before state legislatures. It is less restrictive in that it does not permanently ban the activity (it imposes a five-year moratorium) nor does it make cloning a criminal act (it instead imposed a civil fine). During the five-year sunset period, said the bill's author, cloned animals could be monitored. In the long run, it might be better to "watch and regulate than to totally prohibit human application" (Senate Rules Committee 1997). The law also contains a research clause protecting cell cloning that does not lead to the replication of a human being (see Table 8.1).

The law is restrictive because it limits all forms of reproductive nuclear transfer "from a human cell from whatever the source" to an

TABLE 8.1 State Laws Regulating Cloning, 2001

Provisions	CA	MI	RI	LA	MO	VA
Makes reproductive cloning a criminal act	No	Yes	No	Yes	No	No
Imposes a permanent ban	No[a]	Yes	No[b]	No[a]	Yes[b]	Yes
Limits more than transfer of cloned embryo	No	Yes	No[c]	No[c]	—	Yes
Limits other forms of nuclear transfer	Yes	No	Yes	Yes	Yes	Yes
Contains research protection clause	Yes	Yes	Yes	Yes	No	Yes

[a] Expires in 2003, unless renewed by legislature.
[b] Imposes a permanent ban on state funding.
[c] Forbids cloning or attempting to clone.

enucleated human egg for the purpose of implanting the resulting embryo for pregnancy. This includes embryo cell, fetal cell, and adult cell nuclear transfer. It also includes egg cell nuclear transfer, which is not cloning at all. The broad wording was substituted at the last minute; it is not clear the legislators were aware they had barred more than reproductive SCNT.

Michigan's anticloning law, packaged as four bills, passed the state senate unanimously in April 1998 (Mich. Comp. Laws section 750, 430a[l]; Mich. Comp. Laws section 333.l6274 [5]). More restrictive than California's law, it amends the state penal code to impose a permanent ban on reproductive cloning, without a sunset period. Said state senator Loren Bennett, sponsor of the main bill, about reproductive cloning, "that's wrong today, that's wrong five years from now, that's wrong 100 years from now" (*Detroit News* 1998). It makes reproductive cloning a felony for which the offender could face ten years in prison, a $10 million fine, or both. Persons who violate the law face a license revocation of at least five years and a $10 million fine. Health facilities that violate the law face a $5 million administrative fine. No state funds may be used to attempt human cloning.

The Michigan law goes beyond California's by forbidding any creation of an embryo through SCNT, even if the embryo is not transferred to a woman's uterus (it forbade "the use of human somatic cell nuclear transfer technology to produce an embryo"). It includes a research exemption clause to protect "scientific research or cell-based therapies not specifically prohibited" by the law. Moreover, whether intentionally or not, it targets SCNT only, not embryo cell nuclear transfer, in contrast to California's law that forbids nuclear transfer using a "human cell from whatever the source."

Rhode Island passed a law in 1998 forbidding the use of SCNT to attempt a pregnancy and in twinning to create identical twins by separating the cells of an embryo (R.I. Gen. Laws section 23-16.4-1 et seq.). Its research protection clause allows the cloning of human cells, genes, and tissues that do not result in the "replication of an entire human being." A corporation or other facility violating the law is subject to a $1 million fine, and an individual faces a $250,000 fine. The law has a five-year sunset provision.

Louisiana passed a law in 1999 with virtually the same definition of cloning as California's. For a four-year period it forbids reproductive cloning or attempting to clone, where cloning is defined as "transferring the nucleus from a human cell from whatever source into a human egg from which the nucleus has been removed" for the purpose of reproductive cloning (La. Rev. Stat. Ann. Section 40:1299.36). Its ban on the buying or selling of an "ovum, zygote, embryo, or fetus with the intent to clone a human being" echoes that of Rhode Island. As stated in its research protection clause, the law allows scientific research and cell-based therapies not forbidden in the law. Its penalties are harsher than those in California. Cloning or attempting to clone carries up to a $10 million penalty, ten years in prison "with or without hard labor" or both. The law imposes administrative penalties of up to $10 million for a violating facility or $5 million for an individual violator. Cloning or attempting to clone is unprofessional conduct leading to the permanent revocation of a license. The law forbids the use of state funds to clone or attempt to clone a human being.

Missouri's law, signed by the governor in 1998, is more vague. It bars the use of state funds for research "with respect to" cloning a human person (Mo. Rev. Stat. Section 1.217). It defines cloning broadly as the "replication of" a human person by taking a cell with genetic material and cultivating it through all stages of development to a new human person. This encompasses egg, embryo, and fetal cell nuclear transfer. The law does not have a sunset clause.

Virginia's law, enacted on April 21, 2001, makes it a civil offense to perform human cloning, "implant or attempt to implant" the product of SCNT into a woman's uterus, possess "the product of human cloning," or ship or receive the product of SCNT in order to implant it into a woman's uterus (Code of Virginia Title 32.1, 162.21-162-22; H 2463; S1305). Human cloning is defined as "the creation of or attempt to create a human being by transferring the nucleus from a human cell from whatever source into an oocyte from which the nucleus has been removed." As in California, the Virginia law forbids all forms of nuclear transfer for reproduction, including egg cell nuclear transfer. It does not include research relating to nuclear transfer, however, and includes a research protection clause. It imposes a permanent ban, with a civil penalty of no more than $50,000 for violation.

A second group of laws regulate embryo research and can be interpreted to bar cloning and other innovative reproductive technologies (Andrews 1997; New York State Task Force on Life and the Law 1998, 386–87). As described by Lori Andrews (2000, A-4), twenty-six states have laws regulating fetal or embryo research. Most of these laws were enacted in response to the legalization of abortion in the early 1970s and the initiation of IVF in the early 1980s. Most were on the books at the time of Dolly's birth.

The laws are diverse and have no clear pattern. Ten state laws relate to embryos, and of these ten, one is a minor regulation and nine bar all embryo research. Of these nine, one bars the creation of an embryo for any purpose other than transfer to a woman's uterus for conception and eight bar all research on live conceptuses. Other state laws relate to research on aborted fetuses. The fetal research laws would affect fetal cell nuclear transfer or EG cell studies but probably not SCNT (Andrews 2000, A4-A5). Some bar the buying and selling of embryos. The laws have differing and often vague definitions of the conceptus, fetus, embryo, and fertilization. For example, South Dakota's new law on embryo research defines an embryo as a "living organism of the species Homo sapiens at the earliest stages of development (including the single-celled stage) that is not located in a woman's body" (S.D. section 34-14-20). This definition is problematic because it is unclear whether a single-cell fertilized egg is an organism. Moreover, it is questionable whether the distinction between an embryo in the body and an embryo outside the body is supportable.

When laws are passed for one purpose or within a particular era, it is unclear whether legislative intent or current interpretation applies to today's issues. Moreover, if the laws forbid research on the product of conception, it is possible they do not cover the cloning process because SCNT is arguably experimental only for the egg (Andrews 1997, 24). Reproductive SCNT is analogous to fertilization in that it is a procedure that leads to a cleaving embryo, and the embryo is not itself subject to an intervention. If this is the case, investigators would not be violating an embryo research law if they engaged in reproductive SCNT aimed at a pregnancy and did not manipulate the embryo.

States may also enact new embryo research laws to prevent ES cell and other research. South Dakota's 2000 law forbids research on cells and tissues derived from human embryos. This targets ES cell research by making it a misdemeanor punishable by up to one year in prison or a $1,000 fine to "knowingly conduct nontherapeutic research that subjects a human embryo to substantial risk of injury or death." Because ES cell extraction using current technology destroys the embryo, researchers are forbidden from extracting ES cells. It is possible more states will pass restrictive laws to forbid ES cell research (Stolberg 2001).

Other state laws relate to the practice of ART. As of 1997, thirty-four states had laws related to donor insemination, twenty-two to surrogacy, and five to egg donation (Andrews 1997). These laws define relationships and set forth conditions for engaging in ART practices. For example, after a California physician had used the eggs and embryos of patients in unauthorized ways without patients' consent, California passed two laws. One required physicians to obtain written consent from patients before using gametes for any purpose other than implantation to the patient or patient's spouse. The second made it a crime knowingly to use spermatozoa, eggs, or embryos for purposes other than those specified on the consent form (Angergame and Tierney 1996). These laws would guard against the unauthorized use of human eggs for SCNT experiments if donors have not explicitly consented to this use of their eggs.

The use of state laws to regulate reproductive SCNT has merits and drawbacks in the development of cloning policy. State laws allow the tailoring of provisions to reflect the political culture of each state. They contrast with national legislation, which assumes a degree of homogeneity across the nation. In addition, with their differing histories, cultures, economies, and perceptions of morality, states produce a policy laboratory, where legal variations are initiated and evaluated for enforceability and impact. Laws cover varied facets of cloning such as barring state funding and the sale of eggs for the purpose of cloning. Some states bar reproductive SCNT only; others forbid any kind of nuclear transfer to human eggs. Some make reproductive cloning a crime; others rely on administrative penalties.

In the event that a state law is poorly conceived, its deleterious impact can be limited to a relatively small constituency, the state population. On the other hand, if a law is carefully crafted and successfully implemented, it can serve as a policy model for other states. As Jack Walker has observed, it is not unusual for a "diffusion of innovation" to take place among the states in which some states are national leaders in the adoption of legislation, others are regional leaders, and still others are followers (Walker 1969). This diffusion invites modeling among states, which minimizes a patchwork quilt of unconnected laws and instead produces related laws reflecting common principles and values. An innovator state for restrictions may be California, which was the first to pass an anticloning law and to initiate a zone of proscribed activity ("nuclear transfer from a human cell from whatever the source") that was considered or adopted by other states. Diffusion is furthered when the National Conference for Commissioners on Uniform State Laws, American Bar Association, or other organizations develop model laws for consideration by the states. Although there is no modeling in embryo research law, ART laws provide potential room for diffusion of innovation.

A drawback of state legislation is that the laws may be preempted by federal legislation (Institute of Government and Public Affairs 2001, 29). Moreover, state legislators may be susceptible to quick and poorly drafted legislation. Laws are not helpful if they are immediately outmoded, overbroad, or vague, or if they interfere with values deemed worthy of protection. Such hastily drafted premature laws are difficult to uproot once in place. In barring a technology while it is still hypothetical, a state engages in prior restraint. If a law affects constitutionally protected activities, it may assert an impermissibly chilling effect on research.

Given the difficulties of contesting state embryo research laws in court, it is likely that broad or vague cloning laws will stay on the books indefinitely. To contest a law in civil court, complainants need to show standing and have the financial resources to sustain a suit. Still, courts have struck down state laws that limit research. In the case of *Lifchez v. Hartigan* (735 F. Supp. 1361 [N.D. Ill. 1990]), a federal district court struck down an Illinois abortion law providing that no person may "experiment upon a fetus produced by the fertilization of a human ovum by a human sperm unless such experimentation is therapeutic to the fetus." The law also stated that its provisions were not intended to forbid IVF. Still, the law did interfere with IVF, the court concluded, because techniques in IVF are experimental and are not necessarily therapeutic even though they are done to achieve a pregnancy. Thus, the law interfered with a woman's "cluster of constitutionally protected" reproductive choices that included "the right to submit to a medical procedure that may bring about, rather than prevent, pregnancy." Moreover, by not defining "experimentation" or "therapeutic," the law left researchers and practitioners guessing at the law's meaning. Thus, the law was constitutionally vague, in violation of 5th Amendment due process.

Federal appellate courts also struck down a Louisiana law forbidding nontherapeutic experimentation on fetuses, where the meaning of experimentation was vague (*Margaret S. v. Edwards*, 794 F2d 994 [5th Cir. 1986]) and a Utah statute barring experimentation on live fetuses, where experimentation was not defined (*Jane L. v. Bangerter*, 61 F3d 1493 [1996] [10th Cir.]). In 2000, a federal appeals court struck down an Arizona law barring fetal research on the grounds of vagueness. The court pointed out that the law omitted definitions for "experimentation," "investigation," and other terms (*Forbes v. Napolitano* [9th Cir.], No. 99-D.C. No. CV-96 [29 December 2000]; Crockin 2001, 9). Andrews surmises that embryo research laws would be less susceptible to being overturned because they target research rather than experimental procedures such as IVF (Andrews 2000).

Another drawback of state lawmaking is that it opens the possibility of researchers "shopping" for more congenial states in which to conduct investigations, thereby undercutting a united front against activities deemed undesirable. Laws may also have negative economic consequences for the state if the law causes a "flight" of employees and corporations to other states and puts the state at a disadvantage in the biotechnology field (Institute of Government and Public Affairs 2001, 28). In addition, state lawmaking is less accessible than federal lawmaking. Obtaining transcripts of hearings in state legislative chambers is often difficult, for example, which limits the utility of state legislatures for discussion and public education. State cloning laws are technique specific, which reduces their flexibility in integrating unexpected research developments. They can be both under- and over-inclusive, which is a frailty common to laws designed to control science.

LAWS AND THE CONSTITUTION

The constitutional implications of state (and federal) laws outlawing reproductive SCNT are worthy of further exploration. Laws that target reproductive SCNT may or may not interfere with reproductive liberty and freedom of scientific inquiry.

One position holds that procreative liberty, which is protected under the constitution, includes the right of individuals to have access to reproductive SCNT. For example, John Robertson argues that infertile married couples have the freedom to have "biologically related offspring" and that reproductive SCNT may be the only way some couples can fulfill this freedom. According to Robertson, reproductive cloning is not "radically or essentially different from many current medical and genetic practices" (U.S. Senate, CLHS-SPHS 1997b, 4). If reproductive SCNT is part of procreative liberty, then U.S. Supreme Court cases dealing with birth control and abortion may apply. As the Court said in *Eisenstadt v. Baird* (405 US 438 [1972]), "If the right of privacy means anything, it is the right of the individual, married or single, to be free from unwarranted governmental intrusion into matters so fundamentally affecting a person as the decision whether to bear or beget a child." Arguably, Supreme Court decisions would make reproductive SCNT "part and parcel of a time-honored individual right to control the circumstances and event of reproduction" (Sunstein 1998, 214).

In general, if a law intrudes on a constitutional (fundamental) right, the state needs to show compelling reasons to justify the law, but if a law intrudes on a lesser right, the state needs only to show a rational relationship between the law and its purpose. If reproductive SCNT is part of procreative liberty, then laws barring the technique would be subject to a high level of scrutiny, which places the burden on the government to show it has a compelling interest in enacting the law. It also means the state may regulate only through the least restrictive method. Andrews believes that narrowly crafted anti-cloning laws would pass strict scrutiny because reproductive SCNT poses physical and psychological risks to children and because "our legal system . . . emphatically protects individuality and uniqueness" (Andrews 1997).

Robertson, in contrast, does not believe that with reproductive SCNT the government can show the "high threshold of harm" needed to "justify federal restrictions on family and reproductive decisions" (U.S. Senate, CLHS-SPHS 1997b, 5). This threshold is not met with reproductive SCNT because the proffered harms, at least in 1997, were unsubstantiated. For example, in response to arguments that reproductive SCNT would violate the essence of being human, endanger the child's welfare, and deny the child his or her individuality, Robertson notes there are many views about what it means to be human, and this is not an effective argument in any event. Moreover, the child born through reproductive SCNT will have all the moral and legal rights of other children and there is no evidence that his or her welfare will automatically be impaired. The child will be an individual because she or he is a different person from the person whose genome was used for SCNT. Among other things, the child will have different mitochondrial DNA and will experience a different fetal environment and upbringing from that of the genome donor.

Robertson believes the state could permissibly bar some uses of reproductive SCNT, such as a person cloning one's parent, which would "completely [reverse] the intergenerational meaning of parent and child" (Robertson 1998, 1442). The state could also initiate procedures, such as requiring the somatic cell source to give consent to have his or her genome used for reproductive SCNT or barring the sale of one's DNA for this purpose (Robertson 1998, 1445). In line with U.S. Supreme Court decisions about procreative liberty, the restrictions would be permissible if they did not pose an undue burden on the individual seeking to make reproductive decisions.

Lawrence Tribe, a law professor, also doubts that early arguments against reproductive SCNT are sufficiently strong to justify banning it (Tribe 1998, 224). At the least, he writes, there should be a presumption against a ban. He expresses concern that a ban would "reinforce particular norms about how children ought to be brought into this world" and foster intolerance about unconventional ways of having children.

A second position is that reproductive SCNT is not part of procreative liberty. A key argument here, made by George Annas, Leon Kass, and others, is that reproductive SCNT is not reproduction and therefore does not fall under the protective umbrella of reproductive liberty (U.S. Senate, CLHS-SPHS 1997a, 3; Kass 1997). Andrews also offers that it is "genetic duplication . . . a sort of recycling" (Andrews 1999, 254). If it is not reproduction, it arguably does not fall within the zone of protection recognized by the U.S. Supreme Court and it is not subject to strict scrutiny. Another argument is that Supreme Court rulings establish a right to reproductive liberty related to contraception and abortion but they do not establish an "individual right to procreate by means of new technologies" (Institute of Government and Public Affairs 2001, 23). Even if reproductive SCNT were procreative liberty, it could still be restricted just as, in an analogy, the Supreme Court held that the right to make personal choices about end-of-life decision making does not include the right

to physician-assisted suicide (Sunstein 1998, 216). Those who con-
clude the government may prohibit reproductive SCNT also argue
that concerns about the child's welfare are sufficient to justify limits
on the technique and that there is no compelling reason to use reproductive cloning given the many alternative ways of having children
(Sunstein 1998, 215; U.S. Senate, CLHS-SPHS 1997a, 3).

The constitutional dimensions of laws forbidding egg cell nuclear
transfer or embryo nuclear transfer, both of which are banned in California and would be banned under some bills before the U.S. Congress, are also worthy of exploration. Although not cloning, egg cell
nuclear transfer has been caught up in the zone of banned activity of
some broadly crafted laws (Bonnicksen 1998). If it is barred, the laws
arguably intrude on reproductive liberty by closing a method of
conception for women with inheritable disease passed by their
mitochondria.

It may also be that reproductive SCNT is midway between reproduction and replication and this may prompt the Court to develop
new standards of review. If an anticloning law reached the U.S.
Supreme Court, and the procedure were used safely for animals, the
Court could recognize different levels of scrutiny depending on the
"degree of liberty the [C]ourt finds appropriate for human cloning as
a form of procreation" (Institute of Government and Public Affairs
2001, 25). It could also be the case that a conservative Court would
decline to review judicial challenges to laws banning reproductive
cloning or would issue a terse opinion upholding a contested law.

Laws limiting embryo research or cloning technology also relate
to freedom of scientific inquiry. While the case law is far less extensive in this area than for reproductive liberty, it can also be argued
that scientific inquiry is constitutionally protected. If it is, then the
state must show a compelling interest to ban categories of research.
Exploring the relationship of r-DNA technology and the Constitution, Ira Carmen takes an expansive view of expression, writing that
experimentation is "expressive activity" (Carmen 1985, 40). Still,
inasmuch as experimentation also has a conduct element and the state
has interests in protecting its citizens from dangerous activities, a
legal question should "[ascertain] empirically the nature and likely
consequences of particular investigations" (Carmen 1985, 41). Carmen recommends a two-part assessment in deciding what is permissible expression: "(a) Is the research essentially either a contribution to

the marketplace of ideas or a contribution to some other concern? and (b) If the former, is the research of such species that a rational decisionmaker could consider it hazardous?" (Carmen 1985, 42).

Richard Delgado and David Miller also argue that the early stages of research, where ideas are generated and hypotheses formulated, amount to freedom of thought beyond governmental control (Delgado and Miller 1978, 372). The testing of hypotheses through experimentation, however, can be controlled to protect the public order. Still, because experimentation is "essential to the exposition of scientific ideas, and indispensable as a step to scientific truth," the government may not "suppress activities simply because [it] disapproves of them" (Delgado and Miller, 374, 380). Support for a constitutional link comes from *Meyer v. Nebraska* (262 US 390, 399 [1923]), in which the Supreme Court wrote in dicta that liberty within the meaning of due process includes the right to "engage in any of the common occupations of life, to acquire useful knowledge." Basic research, where the activity is "essential to the generation of new ideas or theories," holds greater constitutional protection than experiments, which may be monitored under the state's police power (Delgado and Miller 1978, 403).

If the Congress were to enact a law barring a whole category of research (SCNT technologies), it would be enacting a content-based prior restraint. Without a compelling reason for imposing this restraint, Congress would appear to be preventing activities because it disapproves of them. Such a law may also violate due process if broadly written. Unconstitutionally vague laws fail to inform people of what is forbidden, lead to arbitrary enforcement, and "inevitably cause people to 'steer far wider of the unlawful zone . . . than if the boundaries of the forbidden areas were clearly marked'" (*Grayned v. Rockford*, 408 US 104 [1972]).

ENABLING REPRODUCTIVE SOMATIC CELL NUCLEAR TRANSFER

It is not out of the question for reproductive SCNT to one day be accepted if safety is established or if attitudes change. The NBAC and other advisory groups recommended that reproductive SCNT should be forbidden with a sunset period of five or more years. California,

Rhode Island, and Louisiana all have sunset clauses in their cloning laws allowing the laws to expire in 2003 unless the legislatures renew them. Robert Oppenheimer notes that new developments such as cloning result in the "obligatory round of chilling scenarios," but the "bitter pill" is not necessarily permanent (Johnson 1997). While opinion polls showed strong public opposition to reproductive cloning in 2000 as well as in 1997 (*Time* Magazine/Cable Network News 2001), a supportive voice is emerging in the scholarly literature and among other commentators (see, e.g., Robertson 1999; Pence 1998; Strong 1998; U.S. House, Committee on Energy and Commerce, Subcommittee on Oversight and Investigations 2001). Laws barring SCNT may not withstand judicial review, new variants of cloning may emerge that fall outside existing laws, and children might be conceived through reproductive SCNT in other nations but born in the United States.

With this variety of contingencies in mind, it is worthwhile to consider the role of the judiciary if reproductive SCNT were to be practiced despite efforts to restrict it. Various relationship questions might arise if reproductive SCNT were clinically available and if involved parties came into conflict. For example, if a married couple were to use the wife's somatic cell to conceive a child through reproductive SCNT and the couple were later to divorce, the woman might claim she should have full custody because she is genetically related to the child while her former husband is not. Or the woman's parents might claim rights over the child because they are, technically, the child's genetic parents. Principles governing such cases would likely emerge in courts, in response to specific conflicts and based on case law developed for assisted conception.

In common law, judges develop principles on a case-by-case basis using actual disputes, and they are guided by analogy and precedent (Dworkin 1996, 7). Such judge-made law holds an appeal in ART cases, where judges wrestle with disputes that many times could not have been anticipated by legislators. For example, an emerging principle in surrogacy disputes is that the persons who intend to be the legal and rearing parents are the ones with prevailing interests (see, e.g., *Johnson v. Calvert*, 851 P2d 776 [1993]; *Marriage of John A. and Luanne H. Buzzanca, In re*, 61 Cal. App. 4th 1410 [1998]). Using this principle, the hypothetical divorced woman mentioned above would presumably have a weak argument against her former husband but a strong argument against her parents. Insofar as the surrogacy cases establish that the parent-child relationship is more than pure genetics and that it involves intentionality, the husband and wife would, in a reasonable scenario, share custody because they together intended to be the child's lawful parents.

The role of common law in enabling novel reproductive technologies is a responsibility not necessarily sought after by judges. Still, as one court wrote, "A child cannot be ignored." No matter what one thinks of surrogacy, cloning, and other conception arrangements, "courts are still going to be faced with the problem of determining lawful parentage" (*Marriage of John A. and Luanne H. Buzzanca, In re*, 61 Cal. App. 4th 1410 [1998]). If a dispute arises about parentage, someone will be called upon to address the relationship, no matter how the child was conceived.

Judge-made law in ARTs has been a default mechanism when state legislators avoid making new laws, despite admonitions by judges who regard ART questions as matters for legislatures rather than courts. Few legislators welcome entering the volatile field of parent-child relationships. There are certain merits of common law, where the capacity to adapt is a source of strength in a time of rapid technological change. Precedent informally carries across jurisdictions, and concurring and dissenting opinions provide a pluralistic voice to troublesome issues. Common law has been a central feature of policymaking in other areas of medicine, such as end-of-life decision making, where patients' rights to end life-sustaining treatment have been established over time and through a mix of state law, judicial cases, legal commentary, and recommendations by advisory bodies. Judge-made law applies "old legal principles to a new technology" in a way that allows for "growth and adaptation" (*Marriage of John A. and Luanne H. Buzzanca, In re*, 61 Cal. App. 4th 1410 [1998]).

On the other hand, common law lacks predictability. It is reactive in that it relies on disputes brought to courts. The process takes a long time, and it is less democratic than legislative action where lawmakers can "formulate general rules based on input from all its constituencies" (*Marriage of John A. and Luanne H. Buzzanca, In re*, 61 Cal. App. 4th 1410 [1998]). Judges are not experts on all issues and are presented with information and arguments from lawyers who are not obligated to present impartial material (Dworkin 1996, 8). Nor do judges have authority over jurisdictions outside their own, so the resolution in one case is not binding on judges in other jurisdictions. When courts do provide frameworks for one another, however, a diffusion of innovation takes place at the judicial level.

CONCLUSIONS

In the area of ARTs and embryo research, state legislatures have generally not provided systematic guidance. This is due in part to the wide variations in laws among the minority of states that have ART, embryo research, and cloning laws. It is also due to laws enacted with political purposes in mind and with little attention to the scientific processes underlying the research in question.

The role of state lawmakers in contributing to the crafting of an overall national cloning policy will depend, in part, on action at the federal level. A federal law forbidding reproductive SCNT would take precedence over less restrictive state laws. It would not, however, preclude the states from enacting laws that are more restrictive, which would give the states a conservative voice. The absence of a federal law would elevate the importance of the states for the citizens of those states with anticloning laws but a patchwork quilt of state laws would not necessarily play a role in national policymaking. It would be more effective for the states to adopt model laws developed by agencies with the resources and skills to develop well-researched model legislation. The National Conference of Commissioners on Uniform State Laws has done this, for example, with the *Uniform Parentage Act*, which has been updated over the years to reflect parenting arrangements that result from assisted conception (National Conference of Commissioners on Uniform State Laws 2000). The adoption of uniform laws across the states brings consistency to state lawmaking. The states also provide a safety net against the irresponsible use of innovative reproductive techniques in clinics through provisions relating to medical malpractice. Licensing restrictions also provide a less onerous method for the states to restrict reproductive SCNT than by making the activity criminal. Just as the federal government has policy channels that are not widely heralded, so too do states have various resources for discouraging reproductive SCNT.

CHAPTER 9

CROSS-NATIONAL AND INTERNATIONAL OVERSIGHT

In examining the U.S. approach to reproductive and therapeutic SCNT, it is helpful to see where the United States stands relative to other nations. Does the U.S. approach fit within or fall outside of cross-national and international norms? How might cloning policies and proposals from other nations inform policymaking in the United States? To address these questions, this chapter examines policy mechanisms in three countries resembling the United States (the United Kingdom, Canada, and Australia), cloning policies in other nations, and recommendations of selected international bodies.

POLICY MECHANISMS IN THE UNITED KINGDOM, CANADA, AND AUSTRALIA

If an examination of policy mechanisms can contribute to the discussion of policy options in the United States, it follows that a look at policies in nations similar to the United States can be especially useful. Although they differ in many ways, three democracies—the United Kingdom, Canada, and Australia—also share a language, cultural heritage, democratic political system, competitive biotechnology industry, and an interest in innovative reproductive technologies. The United Kingdom and Australia in particular are home to pioneering ART research and practices. The governments of all three have experimented with different oversight mechanisms for innovative reproductive technologies.

United Kingdom

The United Kingdom has perhaps the most comprehensive approach for managing innovative reproductive and genetic technologies of all nations in which ARTs are practiced. Its *Human Fertilisation and Embryology Act of 1990* (HFE Act) created a statutory licensing authority, the Human Fertilisation and Embryology Authority (HFEA), to license laboratories working with human embryos and to monitor and set the conditions for embryo research (*International Digest of Health Legislation* [*IDHL*] 1991). The HFEA, the "first statutory body of its type in the world," issues licenses to facilities in which embryos are created, used, or stored (United Kingdom, Human Genetics Advisory Committee [HGAC] 1998b, 5). The authority keeps a registry of licensed research at clinics that use embryos, perform IVF, or store gametes and embryos. It conducts annual inspections of licensed centers and issues an annual report documenting the number of clinics, research projects, and issues raised. The HFE Act distinguishes among ARTs that are illegal (e.g., research beyond fourteen days after fertilization), legal if performed with a license (e.g., creating embryos for research), and unregulated (e.g., gamete intrafallopian tube transfer). The HFEA can suspend or revoke licenses. Conducting research without a license invites criminal sanction.

The HFE Act had its roots in the early 1980s when the United Kingdom, as the home of the first IVF birth in 1978, set up the sixteen-member Committee of Inquiry into Human Fertilisation and Embryology, with Dame Mary Warnock as chair. The committee solicited information from individuals and groups and engaged in deliberations about the ethical dimensions of embryo research and the practice of ARTs. Its outcome, the Warnock Report, made a set of recommendations, including a proposal to establish a national body to issue licenses for embryo research, inspect facilities, and develop a code of practice (Warnock 1985). Eventually the HFE Act was drafted and, after considerable parliamentary debate, passed the House of Lords by a 234 to 80 free vote and the House of Commons by a 364 to 193 free vote. In a separate and nearly identical vote, parliament voted to set up a statutory licensing authority (Warden 1990; Aldous 1990).

The HFEA reviews research protocols under guidelines contained in the Code of Practice and it revisits the code each year in light of changing technologies and practices. The original HFE Act allowed licenses for research using human embryos for five categories of research related to fertility and reproduction:

- promoting advances in the treatment of infertility
- increasing knowledge about the causes of congenital disease
- increasing knowledge about the causes of miscarriage
- developing more effective techniques of contraception
- developing methods for detecting the presence of gene or chromosome abnormalities in embryos before implantation (*IDHL* 1991, 70).

Although the HFEA is the primary apparatus in the United Kingdom for integrating innovative technologies into practice, several other advisory bodies also deliberate and make recommendations. One purpose of the Royal Society, an independent academy of scientists and a funding agency founded in 1660, is to inform policymaking (Royal Society 2001b). It does this by producing reports on issues in science and technology, promoting public awareness of science, and encouraging "innovative scientific research." The Nuffield Council on Bioethics (NCB) is an independent body established in 1991 and funded by the Nuffield Foundation, the Medical Research Council, and the Wellcome Trust. The NCB is a fifteen-member group charged with identifying ethical issues raised by medical research and examining issues to promote public understanding (NCB 2001). It has produced reports on genetically modified crops, genetic screening, human tissue storage, xenotransplantation, and mental disorders and genetics.

At the government level, the Human Genetics Commission (HGC) is a framework for reviewing bioethical issues raised by new genetic technologies (HGC 2000). Beginning its work in late 2000, it is designed to be an independent commission providing guidance on issues related to novel technologies. Its members, who are appointed on the basis of merit, advise the Department of Health, the Office of Science and Technology, and other governmental agencies. The HGC is the fourth of a series of committees; the Advisory Committee on Genetic Testing became the Advisory Group on Scientific Advances in Genetics, which in turn became the Human Genetics Advisory Commission in 1996. The last was changed by administrative act in 1999 to become the HGC.

The British policy for managing innovative technologies, which revolves around the HFEA and the other advisory groups, was called into action for both reproductive and therapeutic SCNT. Public reaction to the birth of Dolly was uniformly negative: Human reproductive SCNT should not proceed. The HFE Act, passed in 1990, had barred licensing for "replacing a nucleus of a cell of an embryo with a nucleus taken from a cell of any person, embryo or subsequent development of an embryo" (*IDHL* 1991, 70; United Kingdom, HGAC 1998b). The language of the act, crafted before reproductive SCNT was remotely possible, left unclear whether reproductive SCNT as well as embryo cell nuclear transfer would be covered. Should the HFE Act be amended to explicitly prohibit reproductive SCNT? Or would the HFEA's discretionary interpretation of the provision suffice?

To consider this issue, the HGAC and the HFEA joined together as a working group, and in January 1998 issued a consultation document on cloning. The document was distributed and members of the public were given three months to respond (United Kingdom, HGAC 1998a). Following consultation with the public, the HGAC and HFEA issued a report in December 1998 advising that the HFE Act did, indeed, forbid licensing for reproductive SCNT and embryo twinning. But, given the seriousness of the issue, the committees called for an explicit ban "enshrined in statute" that would fortify HFEA interpretations (United Kingdom, HGAC 1998b, 2, 4, 9–10). The Science and Technology Committee of the House of Commons also recommended that parliament pass a law explicitly barring human reproductive SCNT. Joining the voices calling for an amendment to the HFE Act, the Royal Society issued a report concluding that reproductive cloning of humans by nuclear substitution was "morally and ethically unacceptable and . . . should be prohibited"

(Royal Society 2001). It sharpened its position in 2001 by calling for an international moratorium on human reproductive cloning (Mayor 2001a).

On July 26, 1997, the minister of state for public health announced that the "deliberate cloning of human beings" would be "ethically unacceptable" and that the HFE Act already barred this activity. Under the act's provisions, he went on, the "cloning of individual humans cannot take place whatever the origin of the material and whatever technique is used" (Masood 1999). Despite the recommendation of the HGAC and HFEA to amend the HFE Act, the government favored using the approach of discretionary interpretation. As of mid-2001, parliament had not specifically outlawed reproductive SCNT, although the government announced it would introduce legislation. Sentiment grew in some quarters for an explicit ban (Mayor 2001a). Policy issues associated with therapeutic SCNT followed closely behind those for reproductive SCNT. As noted above, the HFE Act allowed embryo research for matters relating to infertility, contraception, miscarriages, congenital disorders, and preimplantation genetic diagnosis. This in effect precluded ES cell research, which was aimed at benefiting people with neurological diseases, cancer, diabetes, heart problems, and other medical conditions outside of reproduction. Should the HFE Act be amended to allow embryo research for therapeutic ends unrelated to reproduction?

For this policy issue, key advisory bodies agreed on the merit of amending the HFE Act, starting with the HGAC/HFEA working group that had recommended clarifying the HFE Act to proscribe reproductive SCNT (United Kingdom, HGAC 1998b). Next, the government asked the chief medical officer, Liam Donaldson, to appoint members of what became the Expert Advisory Group (EAG) to consider whether to amend the HFE Act to allow the licensing of ES cell research (Stone 2000). In the meantime, the NCB convened a round table meeting of five people, which produced a discussion paper on stem cell research published on April 16, 2000, and delivered to the EAG (NCB 2000). The NCB recommended that the law be amended to allow embryo research for medical purposes and to allow the creation of new embryos for medical therapies. The EAG, also known as the Donaldson Committee, accepted reports on ES cell research from the NCB and the Royal Society and issued its report in mid-2000 (United Kingdom, Department of Health 2000). With conclusions similar to those of the NCB, the EAG recommended amending the HFE Act to allow embryo research for medical purposes, therapeutic SCNT to produce ES cells, and egg cell nuclear transfer to circumvent mitochondrial diseases (Stone 2000).

The government endorsed the EAG's recommendations in August 2000 and asked Parliament to amend the HFE Act to add three categories of embryo research that could be licensed and that would include ES cell research, even involving embryos generated through SCNT:

- increasing knowledge about the development of embryos
- increasing knowledge about serious disease
- enabling any such knowledge to be applied in developing treatments for serious disease (United Kingdom, HFEA 2001, 3).

In Parliament, the concerns of some members of Parliament (MPs) that therapeutic nuclear transfer would lead to reproductive SCNT joined with long-standing concerns about embryo research in general. Acknowledging the contentious nature of the issue and the personal dilemmas it raised for MPs, the government made the vote in the House of Commons a free vote, which meant MPs were not bound to vote with their party (Vogel 2001a). On December 19, 2000, the House of Commons voted 366 to 174 to amend the law to add categories of research, which, it was understood, would allow licensing for therapeutic SCNT (Dickson 2001).

The politics surrounding the vote were heated. The Campaign Against Human Engineering, the ProLife Alliance, Life, Society for the Protection of the Unborn Child, and other anti-abortion groups argued against the proposal while the Royal Society, Wellcome Trust, Medical Research Council, Roslin Institute, NCB, and other organizations supported it. Organizations associated with specific diseases also argued in favor, including the Parkinson's Disease Society, Diabetes UK, Alzheimer's Society, Huntington Disease Association, British Medical Association, British Heart Foundation, and Cancer Research Campaign (Mayor 2001b). As in the United States, personal testimonies were given, including one by Anne Begg, a Labour MP with Gaucher's disease (Dickson 2001).

On January 22, 2001, the House of Lords voted by an unexpectedly large 120-vote majority to adopt the changes. The Archbishop of Canterbury and other religious leaders had earlier proposed an amendment to send the matter to a Lords select committee before voting on it. This move to postpone failed by a 212 to 92 vote but the Lords accepted an amendment to approve the changes and set up a review committee (Environment News Service 2001). In the meantime, the ProLife Alliance sued the secretary of state for health, arguing that embryos created by nuclear transfer were not created by fertilization and therefore were not embryos under the HFEA (*Nature Biotechnology* 2001). A hearing was scheduled, and the government agreed not to issue licenses before the matter was resolved in the courts. In November 2001, the High Court of Justice ruled that the HFE Act covered only embryos created by the fertilization of an egg by a spermatozoan and not embryos created through SCNT (*Science* 2001c). The Court of Appeal reversed this decision in January 2002, however. The reversal opened the way for research to proceed, and the first licenses to develop ES cell lines from embryos created through SCNT were granted in March 2002 (Mayor 2002).

Canada

Canada, like the United Kingdom and Australia, has a parliamentary political system and, like the United Kingdom, has more of a collectivist than individualistic social and political orientation (Young 1998). Its government has shown a commitment to biotechnology. The Royal Commission on the New Reproductive Technologies provides to Canada a similar source of guiding principles for ARTs and embryo research as did the Warnock Commission in the United Kingdom. In 1989, the government appointed the Royal Commission to examine and report on the implications of the new reproductive technologies. After meeting over a period of fourteen months and soliciting written and oral testimony in a process that ultimately involved over 40,000 participants, the Commission issued in 1993 a two-volume report concluding that embryo research was permissible under specified conditions (Canada, Royal Commission on New Reproductive Technologies 1993). The Royal Commission report identified eight principles to guide decision making and it became an authoritative source on embryo research in the absence of a national law. It favored a "moderate and controlled approach" to innovation and reflected a consensus that a national approach should govern ARTs and embryo research (Natural Sciences Engineering Research

Council of Canada 2001). It favored a regulatory licensing body with subcommittees and it recommended forbidding specific practices, including cloning, animal-human hybrids, gestation outside the uterus, and payment for surrogacy. Later, the Minister of Health called for a voluntary moratorium on nine reproductive and genetic technologies (Marleau 1995). Then, the government introduced Bill C-47, the *Human Reproductive and Genetic Technologies Act*, to parliament in mid-1996. The bill was primarily prohibitive: Among other things, C-47 would have made thirteen practices criminal, including cloning and others covered by the voluntary moratorium. Because bills on the docket are erased in Canada when elections are held, Bill C-47 died when new elections were called in April 1997 (Young 1998).

After the 1997 elections, a member of parliament introduced a private member's bill, C-247, targeting two of the thirteen listed activities from Bill C-47. This new bill would amend the criminal code to proscribe cloning and germ-line alterations:

> No person shall knowingly (a) manipulate an ovum, zygote or embryo for the purpose of producing a zygote or embryo that contains the same genetic information as a living or deceased human being or a zygote, embryo or foetus, or implant in a woman a zygote or embryo so produced; or (b) alter the genetic structure of an ovum, human sperm, zygote or embryo if the altered structure is capable of transmission to a subsequent generation (Canada 1997).

Bill C-247 was referred to the Standing Committee on Health to reconsider the first clause, which some regarded as too broad. Bill C-247, as Bill C-47 before it, died on the docket when new elections were called in 2000.

Efforts to enact a national policy recommenced after the 2000 elections. This time attention turned to a licensing scheme similar to that in the United Kingdom. To encourage public participation, the Policy and Consultation Branch of the Special Projects Division of Health Canada distributed a discussion workbook describing a plan to distinguish between prohibited activities (e.g., reproductive cloning) and regulated activities (e.g., embryo research) and to set up a licensing body (Health Canada, Policy and Consultation Branch [HC-PCB] 2000). The body would be empowered to inspect and license facilities, maintain a central registry, consult with the public, and recommend policy. Reproductive cloning would be a prohibited practice, as would germ-line alterations, research on embryos beyond fourteen days, and other acts held to be unacceptable in the Royal Commission report.

Regulated activities, on the other hand, would be allowed through revocable licenses. The scope of licensing would be broader than under the original HFE Act in the United Kingdom, where embryo research was restricted to studies relating to reproduction. The proposed Canadian plan would allow the use of human gametes or embryos "for research or medical purposes (any procedure for the prevention, diagnosis or treatment of a disease or any other medical condition)" (HC-PCB 2000, 4). A licensing body designed to be flexible, accountable, and transparent would administer the plan (HC-PCB 2000, 11). The body would be developed either internally within Health Canada, a federal department that protects and improves the health of citizens, or externally but still as a part of Health Canada. The mission would be to balance health protection and safety with scientific advances in the public interest (HC-PCB 2000, 10). The Health Minister presented the plan to the Standing Committee on Health of the House of Commons in May 2001, with the request that parliament report back by January 2002.

Among other mechanisms in Canada for assessing innovative reproductive technologies is the recently formed Canadian Institutes of Health Research (CIHR), a network of researchers across the country at thirteen different institutes (CIHR 2001a). Funds are available to researchers in all areas relating to health, including human genetics, and are tied with research protections for human subjects. With CIHR funding, research protections will be developed for human subjects, which will give an opening to heightened oversight for certain categories of research. For example, the CIHR Working Group on Stem Cells Research issued a discussion paper, solicited public responses, and recommended funding for the derivation and use of ES cells for medical purposes with spare embryos (CIHR 2001b). It recommended against the creation of embryos for ES cells and against the creation of embryos through nuclear transfer for therapeutic purposes (CIHR 2001c). Thus, it falls midway between recommendations by advisory groups in the United States and United Kingdom. It also proposed a national oversight body to monitor all privately and publicly funded ES cell research.

Other bodies available to contribute to the debate over innovative technologies are the Royal Society of Canada, which funds research and issues reports, and the National Council on Ethics in Human Research (NCEHR), funded by the Medical Research Council and Health Canada. The NCEHR provides support and information for research ethics boards, which serve similar functions to IRBs in the United States and institutional ethics boards in Australia.

The Canadian Biotechnology Advisory Committee (CBAC) originated with the Canadian Biotechnology Strategy of 1998, which called for public scrutiny of the ethical and environmental features of responsible biotechnology (Industry Canada 1998). The CBAC is an independent panel that advises ministers on the ethical, regulatory, public health, and other aspects of biotechnology; holds public consultations; and produces reports. By mid-2001, it had undertaken five special projects relating to regulation of genetically modified foods, biotechnology and intellectual property, genetic privacy, incorporating societal and ethical considerations into biotechnology, and the use of novel genetically based interventions.

Australia

The state of Victoria in 1979 was "one of the world's leading centers" for IVF, and the country was also the home of the first infant conceived after embryo freezing and thawing. In these and other ways, Australia has been a leader in ART research and practice (Walters 1998, 343). In 1982, in response to a growing number of IVF births in the state of Victoria, the Victorian government appointed the Committee to Consider the Social, Ethical and Legal Issues Arising from *In Vitro* Fertilization, chaired by Louis Waller. The Waller Committee issued three reports to advise policymakers, and it contributed to deliberations on how to monitor developments in embryo research and reproductive technologies (Walters 1998, 343). The Waller Report provided guidance for Australia similar to that provided by the Warnock Committee for the United Kingdom and the Royal Commission for Canada.

Australia has a federal system of government made up of two territories and six states. Over time, Australian embryo research policy has taken the form of national guidelines applicable to all but three states, which have enacted their own laws. Two sets of guidelines for

ARTs prevail at the national level. One governs all public human subjects research and, among other things, sets out the conditions for institutional ethics committees. The other, the 1996 National Health
and Medical Research Council (NHMRC) Ethical Guidelines on Assisted Reproductive Technology, guides embryo research and ARTs
in particular (Australian Academy of Science 2001, 18). Section 6.4 of
the NHMRC guidelines allows institutional ethics committees to approve embryo research "in exceptional circumstances" where there is
the "likelihood of a significant advance in knowledge or improvement
in technologies for treatment" (p. 19). Section 11.1 provides that no
embryos may be created for research purposes. Publicly funded researchers use these guidelines, and privately funded investigators are
invited to follow them (CIHR 2001b, 15).

Three Australian states have embryo research laws that preempt
the national guidelines. The state of Victoria passed the *Infertility
(Medical Procedures) Act of 1984*, which created a Standing Review and
Policy Committee to review embryo research. In 1995, Victoria re-
placed the 1984 act with a restrictive law, the *Infertility Treatment Act
of 1995*, that makes research even on spare embryos a criminal act
(Brody 1998, 112–13; Australian Academy of Science 2001, 20). Even
so, it does allow research on ES cells derived elsewhere and imported
into the country. Western Australia and South Australia have licensing laws for embryo research that permit embryo research under
strict conditions. Because state laws prevail over national guidelines,
Australian law on embryo research is not uniform (Australian Academy of Science 2001, 20, 22).

On the matter of reproductive and therapeutic SCNT, the minister for health and aged care asked the Australian Health Ethics
Council (AHEC) to issue an advisory report on human reproductive
cloning, which was published in late 1998 (AHEC 1998). The AHEC
noted that human cloning was barred in the three states and precluded by the 1996 NHMRC guidelines, which did not allow funding
for "experimentation with the intent to produce two or more genetically identical individuals, including development of human embry-
onal stem cell lines with the aim of producing a clone of individuals."
The council recommended that all states and territories in Australia
allow only embryo research permitted in the NHMRC's guidelines.
The minister gave the report to a standing committee in the House

of Representatives, which in turn commenced an inquiry into human cloning.

In the meantime, the Australian Academy of Science published a report recommending that the 1996 NHMRC guidelines be amended to permit therapeutic SCNT and that some restrictive state legislation be repealed (Australian Academy of Science 2001, 33). The academy recommended initiating a national two-tiered review process that would be binding on private and public researchers and that would bring consistency to the nation's policy. The plan would involve local review of embryo research protocols and then review by a national panel set up by the NHMRC. The framework would limit some research such as cloning but it would not "regulate the details of research practice" (Australian Academy of Science 2001, 20).

In an additional cloning development, in late December 2000, the Australian parliament passed the *Gene Technology Act*. This law dealt with genetically modified crops, but it contained a provision barring funding for studies to create "a duplicate or descendant that is identical to the original" human (Australian Academy of Science 2001, 23).

At the state level, the embryo research laws of Western Australia, Victoria, and South Australia outlaw reproductive cloning. For example, Western Australia's law of 1991 stipulates that "human cloning" or the replacement of the nucleus from an egg or embryo in the process of fertilization is not allowed under penalty of a fine or imprisonment. A fourth state, New South Wales, issued a discussion paper in 1997, "Review of the Human Tissue Act of 1983," stating the government's intention to forbid human cloning and cross-species fertilization (Eiseman 2000, 164).

Observations

Several observations can be made about policies in the United Kingdom, Canada, Australia, and the United States. First, as of 2001, the United Kingdom was the only one of these four nations to have a comprehensive regulatory mechanism governing embryo research and, with it, a framework for managing innovative technologies. This mechanism has a clear history, with the Warnock Report, HFE Act, and HFEA initiated sequentially. The HFEA is flexible, and licensing for embryo research is a matter of public record. As the chair of the HFEA said of the structure in 2001, "There is a clear framework, there are layers of enforceability starting with the primary legislation going through regulations, directions, and a code of practice, which have meant that we have been able to oversee progress on the medical and scientific fronts in a responsible and controlled manner" (Grubb 2001, 6, quoting Ruth Deech). Adding to this central oversight mechanism are the NCB, Royal Society, and HGC, all of which contribute to the public examination of issues relating to innovative technologies.

Although Australia does not have a national licensing system on the order of the United Kingdom's, its 1996 NHMRC guidelines provide national-level guidance for managing innovation. This provides a structure around which to orient discussions when innovative research is proposed and policy modifications are debated. Even though the laws of three states preempt the guidelines, the NHMRC rules still provide a set of principles from which deliberations can proceed. Canada and the United States lack even this degree of national oversight, but Canada has two things that the United States lacks: a respected document of principles and guidelines developed over time through a democratic procedure (the Royal Commission report) and a comprehensive plan for a licensing system in process. If Canada's plan is implemented, this will leave the United States as the most laissez-faire of these four nations.

Second, all four nations place a value on deliberative processes and public debate. In each, policymaking is a slow, incremental, and cautious procedure with multiple private and public advisory bodies. There is consensus that reproductive SCNT should not proceed, but with variations in how this is implemented. Policymakers in all these nations are grappling with similar issues involving ES cells, such as whether therapeutic SCNT should be allowed and/or funded. Evidence that advisory groups in one nation refer to position statements by advisory groups in another suggests the viability of an international modeling or diffusion of innovation.

Third, the nations have different contextual constraints. Differing perspectives on the status of the embryo and fetus significantly color the nature of debates over embryo research in the United States. The matter is not as divisive in Australia and Canada, but it does influence policy deliberations in the United Kingdom. For example, pro-life groups mounted vigorous dissent over whether to amend the HFE Act to permit ES cell research in 2000. Religious leaders representing the Anglican and Roman Catholic churches, the chief rabbi, and the president of the Muslim College also protested and urged a delay in the parliamentary vote (Mayor 2001b). Religious and pro-life groups also asserted a powerful voice when the HFE Act was debated in 1989–1990. The disputes have not been of sufficient intensity to prevent permissive embryo research policies, however.

While the United Kingdom enjoys some things that facilitate innovative policy, it has a contextual influence not felt in Canada, Australia, or the United States, namely, the harmonization efforts of the European Union and the integration of the European Convention on Human Rights (Bahadur 2001). For example, in advance of the British vote on the measure to allow therapeutic SCNT, the European Parliament passed a resolution by a 237–230 vote (with forty abstentions) stating that "'therapeutic cloning,' which involves the creation of human embryos purely for research purposes, . . . crosses a boundary in research norms" (European Parliament 2000). The European Parliament also sent a letter signed by fifty-eight members urging that a select committee be appointed to study the matter further (ProLife Alliance 2001). Still, inasmuch as the U.K. government proceeded on its vote, this constraint was not determinative.

The similarities among these nations in their procedural respect for open deliberation and the shared timeliness of issues involving ES cell research, therapeutic SCNT, and reproductive SCNT point to the value of trying to build cross-national governing principles. The impetus for this may be fostered by cross-national research collaborations that involve movement of researchers as well as ideas (*Science* 2001a).

POLICIES IN OTHER NATIONS
Embryo Research and Cloning Laws

In a survey of national policies on embryo research and ARTs, Howard W. Jones, Jr., and Jean Cohen distinguished between "framework" nations with national laws and "guideline" nations with principles and rules developed by commissions and professional associations (Jones and Cohen 1999). Among the member states of the European Union, only Germany has a law specifically crafted for embryo research; six nations regulate embryo research within ART laws

(Austria, Denmark, France, Spain, Sweden, and United Kingdom); and the remaining nations have no laws directly relating to embryo research. The laws use different definitions of the embryo, which diminishes the ability to draw generalizations. Early in the twenty-first century, five nations were drafting legislation specific for embryo research (Belgium), for inclusion in ART laws (Italy, The Netherlands, and Portugal), or for inclusion in provisions about medical research (Finland) (European Commission, EGE 1999, 126).

In the matter of reproductive cloning, only a handful of the world's nations have laws with cloning provisions. Several nations had laws with anticloning provisions before Dolly's birth, including Australia, Austria, Denmark, France, Germany, Norway, Slovakia, Spain, Switzerland, and the United Kingdom (Eiseman 2000, 164). Three added anticloning laws after Dolly's birth (Israel, Malaysia, and Peru), and at least six have proposed laws (Argentina, Belgium, Canada, China, Japan, and South Korea). Jones and Cohen's survey of thirty-eight nations revealed that nineteen barred human reproductive cloning by law, thirteen had guidelines for practitioners to follow, and six had neither laws nor guidelines for reproductive cloning (Jones and Cohen 1999, 28S).

In most cases, anticloning prohibitions appear in embryo research and ART laws. Under Germany's *Embryo Protection Act of 1990*, cloning by embryo or fetal or adult SCNT is a criminal offense, resulting in a prison term of up to five years or a fine (*Human Reproduction* 1991). The law is generally prohibitive in other ways as well. It makes misuse of human embryos a criminal act, where misuse is buying or acquiring a human embryo "for purposes other than preserving its development" or allowing an embryo to develop "for purposes other than causing a pregnancy." It defines the embryo as a fertilized human egg, including "any totipotent parts" that could develop into an individual being, and it thus makes each undifferentiated embryo cell a human being (*Human Reproduction* 1991). This outlaws preimplantation genetic diagnosis, in which a cell of the early embryo is removed for DNA amplification and testing.

Austria also has a restrictive embryo research law that forbids the donation of eggs and embryos for research (CIHR 2001b, 14). Denmark's biomedical research law of 1992 makes it illegal to produce individuals who are genetically identical, and it forbids nuclear transfer (Eiseman 2000, 165). In 2001, however, the Danish Council of Ethics recommended to the Danish parliament that therapeutic cloning be allowed if no embryos were created solely for research (Skovmand 2001). France's embryo research law, as interpreted through decrees, forbids interventions that would adversely affect the embryo's "developmental capacities" (*IDHL* 1997b). It allows experimentation if the procedure is therapeutic and the embryo will be transferred to a woman's uterus. France's bioethics laws of 1994 (Law 94-653 and Law 94-654) forbid human cloning, but the French National Bioethics Committee recommended that the ban be made more explicit when the bioethics law was revised in 1999 (United Kingdom, HGAC 1998b, 35). Deliberations are underway about whether to change the 1994 law to allow ES cell research using spare embryos with the consent of donors (Normile 2000). The proposal would allow the derivation of ES cells from seven- to twelve-day embryos donated from IVF programs under the oversight of an eighteen-member panel, but it would maintain the ban on reproductive cloning (Reuters 2000).

The Spanish law on ARTs disallows the fertilization of eggs for purposes other than reproduction and it attaches criminal penalties to embryo cloning (*IDHL* 1999). Norwegian law implicitly bars cloning by prohibiting research on fertilized eggs. This law would include cloning in its experimental stages but it would not necessarily forbid reproductive SCNT if the technique were safe. Thus, Norway's parliament passed an additional law explicitly banning the cloning of humans and "highly developed organisms" (Voelker 1997). Slovakia's 1994 Health Care Law implicitly forbids reproductive SCNT, as does Sweden's Law 115 of 1991. Switzerland's Law on Reproductive Medicine in Humans (1990) bars embryo research, cloning, animal-human hybrids, extracorporeal gestation, chimeras, and germ-line gene therapy, and the federal constitution also forbids embryo cloning (Eiseman 2000, 166; United Kingdom, HGAC 1998b, 35–36).

Few nations outside the Anglo nations and Europe have enacted embryo research, ART, or cloning laws. A survey in the mid-1990s revealed that of sixteen Asian and Middle Eastern nations contacted, only Taiwan had legislation directed to ARTs (Schenker and Shushan 1996). Since this survey was conducted, Malaysia passed a law barring reproductive cloning, as did Peru (Eiseman 2000, 167). In 1998, the Israeli Knesset passed a five-year moratorium on reproductive cloning, with a two-year prison term for violators, but it authorized the health minister to allow cloning if it could be done without violating human dignity (Israeli Knesset 1998). In 1997, China's health minister said the government opposed human reproductive cloning and said scientists should not participate in research to clone human beings (Normile 2000; Eiseman 2000, 168).

In Japan, the Council for Science and Technology proposed banning human cloning and preparing guidelines for research using cloned embryos (*Nature* 1999b). In 2001, guidelines were proposed allowing basic ES cell research that would allow reproduction or the development of medical therapies (Normile 2001). A 1997 decree in Argentina prohibited "cloning experiments involving human beings" and required the Ministry of Health and Social Action to formulate a draft law (*IDHL* 1997a).

Observations

Several observations can be made about cloning policies among nations. Many of the nations with advanced scientific infrastructures have laws or policies to preclude reproductive cloning. Taken overall, however, few of the world's nations have cloning laws. The absence of laws in countries without advanced biotechnology capacities would potentially allow scientists from industrial nations to conduct research in nations without such laws. For nations without laws or for which cloning is of low legislative priority, international documents such as the declaration by the United Nations Educational, Scientific, and Cultural Organization (UNESCO), discussed below, provide guiding principles.

A great degree of pluralism exists across nations due to such things as embryo research policies, tolerance for ambiguity, and methods for grappling with bioethical controversies in general (Byk 1994). In 1998, the European Community (EC) asked the EGE to prepare a report to help the EC make decisions about funding programs. Reviewing the laws and approaches of the EC's member states toward the human embryo, the EGE observed that the extreme differences made it "difficult to see how . . . the differences can be reconciled" (European Commission, EGE 1999, 128). Bowing to this diversity, the EGE concluded it would be "inappropriate to impose one exclusive moral code" about embryo research on the member states.

Moreover, respecting moral and legal diversity is part of the ethic behind the European Union, the EGE wrote, and it is "essential to the building of Europe."

The EGE recommended that the Fifth Research Framework Programme, which had proposed withholding funding for any project involving the destruction of human embryos, "should not a priori exclude European financial support for human embryo research carried out in countries where it is permitted" (European Commission Secretariat-General 1998). Nevertheless, the Framework Programme should give "particular attention" to ethical issues in research in the "most sensitive fields" and give high priority to respect for human life. For Fifth Research Framework funding to be allowed, embryo research should be conducted under "strict public control" with "maximum transparency" (European Commission, EGE 1999, 128). The divisiveness of the embryo research issue is evidenced by the fact that about one-half of the EGE's opinions relate to embryo research (Lenoir 2000, 1426). Noelle Lenoir, chair of UNESCO's International Bioethics Committee, has concluded that no single standard on embryo research can be expected.

National laws are individually tailored, although agreements in the Council of Europe, discussed below, place a premium on harmonized laws. Many are in flux as a result of issues similar to those besetting the United States. The issues raised by ES cell research challenge policymakers in France, Switzerland, Germany, and other nations to determine whether to carve exceptions in embryo research laws to accommodate ES cell research, allow therapeutic SCNT, and/or allow the import of ES cells for researchers' use (*Nature* 2001; *Science* 2001b; Schiermeier 2001).

Nevertheless, some principles about embryo research draw consensus across European nations that allow embryo research. Among these nations it is generally agreed that embryos will not be studied for more than fourteen days after fertilization, research embryos will not be transferred for pregnancy; gamete providers will give consent before research is conducted on gametes or embryos; embryos will not be generated for research, embryos will not be bought or sold; embryos will not be genetically modified; and human-animal hybrids will not be created (European Commission, EGE 1999, 126–27; Lenoir 2000, 1425). Values common across Europe embrace respect for human life, relief of suffering, safe medical treatment, freedom of research, and informed consent. In addition, a recurring principle in European discussions is that the human genome is a collective good that represents "the collective assets of a community," has "enduring worth," and deserves protection. Because reproductive cloning, if widely practiced, could affect genetic diversity (Eisenberg 1999), limiting it could be justified as a way of protecting the genome as a shared resource. The principle of the genome as a collective resource is widely but not universally accepted in Europe. It highlights the principle of distributive justice in assessing the desirability of novel technologies.

INTERNATIONAL RESPONSES TO REPRODUCTIVE CLONING

Nongovernmental Organizations

International organizations and associations at both the governmental and nongovernmental levels provide a barometer of sentiment about novel reproductive and genetic technologies. For reproductive cloning, the sentiment at the nongovernmental level was overwhelmingly negative as professional organizations and associations quickly distanced themselves from the idea of cloning. For scientists and medical professionals, reproductive cloning did not pass ethical muster, at least at present, and most regarded moral persuasion as the preferred method over banning to prevent reproductive cloning. Professional societies linked to infertility treatment and reproductive biology issued cautionary statements about reproductive cloning. For example, the European Society for Human Reproduction and Embryology in 1997 called for a five-year moratorium on reproductive SCNT. It reaffirmed this position in 1999 when it indicated support of therapeutic SCNT (*Nature* 1999a).

The Executive Council of the World Medical Association, which represents seventy medical associations, urged physicians and researchers in 1997 to voluntarily abstain from human cloning "until the scientific, ethical and legal issues have been fully considered by doctors and scientists and any necessary controls put in place" (Reuters 1997). The Ethical, Legal and Social Issues Committee of the Human Genome Organisation (HUGO) issued a statement on cloning after Dolly's birth that said there "should be no attempt to produce a genetic 'copy' of an existing human being by somatic cell nuclear transfer" (HUGO Ethics Committee 1999). The statement pointed out the different uses to which SCNT could be put and it warned against interfering with basic research on SCNT. Such research could lead to benefits, including therapeutic interventions and the avoidance of diseases linked to mutations in mitochondrial DNA. The HUGO Ethics Committee recommended that in the course of studying therapeutic SCNT, researchers should not allow in utero development of embryos created through SCNT. It reiterated principles from the committee's Statement on the Principled Conduct of Genetics Research, which considered the human genome to be "part of the common heritage of humanity." Balanced against the pursuit of scientific research must be respect for "international norms of human rights," a recognition of the "values, traditions, culture, and integrity of participants," and the need to uphold "human dignity and freedom" (HUGO 1996; Lenoir 1997). The Committee also acknowledged the widespread unease about the deliberate creation of embryos for research.

One of the science-oriented organizations that called for a ban on cloning was the Council for Responsible Genetics, a group formed out of concern for the social implications of genetic engineering. In a cloning paper issued in 1997, it called upon all nations to incorporate prohibitions against cloning humans in their laws and it urged the United Nations to create a forum to express concerns about human cloning (Council for Responsible Genetics 1997).

Governmental Organizations

Shortly after Dolly's announced birth, the director general of the World Health Organization (WHO), a group with 191 member nations and including the United States, condemned human cloning as contrary to the respect accorded the human being. Two months later, members attending the WHO's fiftieth session of the World Health Assembly resolved that "the use of cloning for the replication of human individuals is ethically unacceptable and contrary to human integrity and morality" (Australian Academy of Science 1999, 27). In 1998, the fifty-first session of the World Health Assembly reaffirmed the 1997 resolution and began drafting a document of guiding principles for health and cloning that would extend beyond reproductive cloning (WHO 1998b; WHO 1999). It raised objections about reproductive cloning, most significantly that it is "ethically unacceptable," and "that it would be contrary to human dignity as it would violate the uniqueness and indeterminateness of the human being" (WHO 1998a). In 2000, the director general called for continued examination of bioethics as a whole (WHO 2000).

Before cloning's debut as an international issue, a UNESCO bioethics committee had begun crafting the Universal Declaration on the Human Genome and Human Rights. It had aimed to complete the document in time for the 1998 celebration of the fiftieth anniversary of the United Nations Declaration of Human Rights. The goal was to balance the values of scientific advance with those of human rights.

The cloning issue posed unexpected challenges for the framers, who had been working on the document for two years. While the framers intended the declaration to be principle based rather than technique based, some nations in the wake of Dolly's birth pressed to list specific techniques that should not be practiced, including germline genetic interventions and reproductive cloning. Faced with the prospect of stalemate over what had been lauded as UNESCO's most significant document, those supporting the original drafts eventually reached a compromise with those who wanted to list proscribed techniques. In the final document, one technique—cloning—was mentioned by name; Article 11 declared that "practices . . . contrary to human dignity, such as the reproductive cloning of human beings, shall not be permitted." This negotiated addition did not define cloning or explain how and why cloning was contrary to human dignity.

UNESCO's 186 member nations unanimously adopted and signed the declaration in November 1997 (UNESCO, International Bioethics Committee 1997). The United States helped draft the declaration, but because the United States was not a member of UNESCO, it did not sign the declaration even though it could have done so. In November 1998, the eighty-six members of the U.N. Commission on Human Rights approved the declaration and the next month the U.N. General Assembly adopted it (Eiseman 2000, 170). The declaration does not legally bind its signatories but it does provide a way for nations without genetic and ART laws to endorse certain principles of human rights.

Of the regional governmental bodies that have deliberated on reproductive cloning, the Council of Europe, with forty member states, has been the most active. The Council of Europe was established in 1949 to promote cooperation among nations. Its Parliamentary Assembly, as the Council's "leading conscience," formulates resolutions and recommendations relating to bioethics (Byk 1994). At one point, the Parliamentary Assembly recommended that the Council recognize a right to a genetic inheritance that has not been artificially changed and seek a transnational harmonization of genetic principles. In response, the Council convened the Bioethics Convention in 1991 to create a legally binding instrument based on principles relative to human rights. It was intended to guide national legislation, reflect differing cultures and legal systems, accommodate rapid technological change, and address public fears about genetics (Wachter 1997).

The resulting document, the Convention for the Protection of Human Rights and Dignity with Regard to the Application of Biology and Medicine, related to genetics rather than cloning, although conceivably an article barring germ-line genetic interventions could cover cloning:

> An intervention seeking to modify the human genome may be undertaken . . . only if its aim is not to introduce any modification in the genome of any descendants (Article 13).

The convention was opened for the signature of the Council's member states on April 4, 1997 (European Commission, EGE 1999, 123). Signing the convention legally obligated member states to bring their own laws into conformity with the convention's principles, unless they attached a reservation relating to articles covered by existing laws (Dommel and Alexander 1997). Twenty-one of the forty member states signed on that date. By February 2000, twenty-eight member states had signed the convention, and the governments of six had ratified it: Denmark, Greece, San Marino, Slovakia, Slovenia, and Spain (Schiermeier 1999, 332). As of 2000, Germany and the United Kingdom had not signed it. Germany resisted the convention's acceptance of research on incapacitated persons, which was forbidden in Germany (Schiermeier 1999, 331). The British resisted restrictions on embryo research that went beyond those in the United

Kingdom. The United States participated in the negotiations; as an observer state, it could sign but it elected not to do so.

In October 1997, after reproductive cloning became an issue, the Council's member states held a summit in Strasbourg. At this meeting, the participants unanimously recommended that member states "undertake to prohibit all use of cloning techniques aimed at creating genetically identical human beings." They also urged the Committee of Ministers to adopt an additional protocol on cloning "as soon as possible" (*IDHL* 1998, 9). The Council of Europe then developed a cloning protocol (Additional Protocol to the Convention for the Protection of Human Rights and Dignity of the Human Being with Regard to the Application of Biology and Medicine, on the Prohibition of Cloning Human Beings). It was opened in early 1998 for the signatures of the member states that had designed the original convention (Council of Europe 1998). Article 1 prohibited "any intervention to create a human being genetically identical to another human being, whether living or dead." It interpreted a "human being 'genetically identical' to another human being" to mean "a human being sharing with another the same nuclear gene set." Nineteen members signed in January 1998. Five nations needed to ratify the protocol for it to come into effect; this occurred in March 2001 (Skovmand 2001).

The European Parliament also joined in the condemnation of cloning. On March 12, 1997, it resolved that cloning was a "serious violation of fundamental human rights." It "permit[s] a eugenic and racist selection of the human race, it offends against human dignity and it requires experimentation on humans" (*IDHL* 1997c, 440). The Parliament urged "an explicit worldwide ban on the cloning of human beings," and it advised member states to "ban the cloning of human beings at all stages of formation and development, regardless of the method used, and to provide for penal sanctions to deal with any violation." The European Parliament had previously deliberated on beginning of life technologies. Its Parliamentary Assembly issued a resolution on genetic engineering in 1989 and a resolution on the cloning of embryos in 1993. The Parliament had also identified global principles, including the "right of a person to his or her own genetic identity" and the "absolute priority for the protection of the dignity and rights of individuals" over the interests of "any social or third party" (*IDHL* 1997c, 440).

The Group of Advisers on the Ethical Implications of Biotechnology of the EC, which later became the EGE, was founded in 1991 to guide the EC on matters involving countervailing values about technological progress and ethics (European Commission Secretariat-General 1998). It issued a report on cloning in 1997 that distinguished among different types of cloning and between reproductive and therapeutic cloning. It recommended prohibiting embryo splitting, embryo cell nuclear transfer, and reproductive SCNT. It encouraged the EC to "clearly express its condemnation of human reproductive cloning" and to act accordingly when making decisions about research funding and patent policy. The European Commission later issued the Directive on the Legal Protection of Biotechnological Inventions, which forbade issuing patents to clone human beings (United Kingdom, HGAC 1998b, 40).

Two articles in the Council of Europe's Bioethics Convention relate to embryos. Article 18.1 states that "where the law allows research on embryos in vitro, it shall ensure adequate protection of the embryo." Article 18.2 forbids the creation of embryos for research among signatory nations. A nation can sign the convention with a reservation, which means a previously drawn law prevails over a particular article. The United Kingdom placed a reservation on Article 18.2 because U.K. law allows the generation of embryos for research under specified conditions. As a result of these objections to Article 18.2, the convention's framers added Article 18.1, as stated above (Brody 1998, 112; European Commission, EGE 1999, 126). Embryos are also protected by a European Commission directive of 1998 barring the patenting of commercial uses of human embryos (European Commission, EGE 1999, 126).

In 2000, the president of the European Commission asked the EGE to prepare a report on therapeutic SCNT and embryo research, and the EGE, chaired by Nicole Lenoir, issued a report on November 14, 2000 (European Commission, EGE 2000; Dickson 2000). The report acknowledged that each member state makes independent decisions about embryo research. Group members held three different positions that reflected viewpoints elsewhere in the embryo research debate: (1) outlaw all embryo research, (2) permit research on spare embryos only, and (3) allow the creation of embryos for research under a controlled regulatory structure. On the matter of therapeutic SCNT, the group urged "prudence" and said the creation of embryos by SCNT for therapeutic research would be "premature."

Using a precautionary approach, the EGE weighed the risks and benefits of embryo research using SCNT. It regarded the benefits as remote in relation to the risks of making embryos trivial and pressuring women to donate oocytes for embryo creation (European Commission, EGE 2000, 17). It pointed out that therapeutic SCNT could pave the way for reproductive SCNT, and it cautioned that if embryos created through SCNT were transferred to a woman's uterus, this would violate European Commission law (p. 10). The report was designed to guide the Fifth Research Framework Programme, but it was also aimed at the United Kingdom, France, and other nations deliberating on therapeutic SCNT.

Among the many agencies and groups that have examined reproductive cloning, UNESCO, Council of Europe, EGE, and European Parliament have all concluded it would be unethical to proceed with the technology. It is not always clear from the statements of these and other groups whether the injunction should be temporary or permanent and whether it should extend to forms of cloning beyond reproductive SCNT (e.g., embryo cell nuclear transfer and twinning). The debate in many ways is in its infancy.

International organizations differ from national governments in the nature of their reservations about cloning. While many national governments craft technique-specific laws, international groups work with documents that focus on principles that would apply to all novel reproductive technologies rather than on technique-specific admonitions. This arguably gives the documents greater lasting power than if they were dependent on stated techniques (Knoppers 1997).

CONCLUSIONS

How important is international sentiment in developing U.S. cloning policy? Looking to different political cultures and systems invites a wider perspective in policymaking and encourages a sense of responsibility to inquire into and acknowledge international mores. While there is no legal obligation to take international sentiment into account, acknowledging that sentiment, even if it is mixed, is a responsible act. If policies in the United States diverge markedly from expectations elsewhere, some justification seems appropriate. Conversely, if policies are consistent with international expectations, they gain credibility and support.

International sentiment can be acknowledged in various ways. One is for policymakers to declare their shared interests publicly. This happened, for example, when leaders from eight major industrial countries agreed in 1997 to work together to strengthen democracy and human rights. The communique issued on behalf of the leaders, of whom President Bill Clinton was one, contained ninety provisions, including No. 47: "We agree on the need for appropriate domestic measures and close international cooperation to prohibit the use of somatic cell nuclear transfer to create a child" (European Commission 1997). Members of the U.S. Congress also acknowledge international interests when they insert into cloning bills references to international relations. For example, H.R. 1644, the *Human Cloning Prohibition Act of 2001*, referred to international condemnation of cloning expressed in the Cloning Protocol of the Council of Europe (U.S. House 2001a). In some bills, the sponsors also call for international cooperation to monitor and police reproductive cloning.

A second method is for advisory bodies to integrate guidelines from other nations into their deliberations. For example, when developing its stem cell advisory document, the NCB adopted NBAC recommendations for securing informed consent to donate embryos for ES cell research (NCB 2000). Advisory bodies also give an international cast to their deliberations when they summarize conclusions reached by bodies in other nations and then distinguish their own recommendations from or build on the earlier reports. At the nongovernmental level, a diffusion of innovation can take place among national, regional, and international fertility societies (e.g., the ASRM, European Society of Human Reproduction and Embryology, and International Federation of Fertility Societies).

The United States is not alone in having minimal policies for embryo research in general and in reproductive SCNT in particular. It is unusual among nations similar to it, however, for not having a national-level forum in place to explore the problematic dimensions of new reproductive technologies. The NBAC did fulfill that role with its report on reproductive SCNT in 1997, which was the first in the world that systematically examined issues related to reproductive SCNT, but the NBAC has since been disbanded. The PCB will provide a new forum for discussing the ethical dimensions of new technologies, but it, as the NBAC before it, is a temporary body appointed by the president. In the United States a minimal national forum and funding restrictions reduce the ability to effectively monitor ongoing research and provide policy leadership.

CHAPTER 10

TOWARD RESPONSIBLE POLICYMAKING

Dolly's birth, which defied an earlier prediction that "the cloning of mammals, by simple nuclear transfer, is biologically impossible," was of exquisite interest to some and of troubling interest to others (McLaren 2000, 480, quoting Davor Solter). Riveting world-wide public attention, the event prompted one science writer to observe that "when the time comes to write the history of our age, this quiet birth, the creation of this little lamb, will stand out" (Kolata 1998a, 2). With the birth came a sense of urgency to ensure that reproductive SCNT would never be used with humans. What does the current study say about our ability to manage this and future innovative technologies?

FOUR POLICY APPROACHES

A coherent policy embraces rules and laws, a vision, and expectations and norms from the private and public sectors (Frankel 2000). It can take many forms (Knoppers, Hirtle, and Glass 1999). In the area of reproductive SCNT, four approaches, not mutually exclusive, have attracted attention: (1) legislation with a narrow arc, (2) legislation with a broad arc, (3) existing regulatory mechanisms, and (4) regulatory mechanisms with adjustments. The depth of concern about cloning, beliefs about the nature of human embryos, attitudes about regulation of biotechnology generally, and trust in the ability of policymakers to draw lines all affect policy preferences. One can surmise that an individual who (1) believes reproductive SCNT poses serious risks to society, (2) imbues the embryo with the status of a person, and (3) distrusts the societal ability to draw lines will be more likely to favor legislation with a broad arc. Conversely, a person who believes the embryo has a lesser status, accepts the ability of policymakers to draw lines, and avers that cloning does not pose extraordinary risks will be more likely to favor existing mechanisms, with or without refinements.

Legislation with a Narrow Arc

Members of Congress have devoted considerable effort to orienting policy around legislation that would narrowly forbid reproductive SCNT. The first bills in 1997 generally would make criminal the cloning of a human being. By 2001, the bills added more careful language to bar more specifically the transfer of an embryo created through SCNT to a woman's uterus. Professional associations and other groups both within and outside the United States have publicly supported this type of bottom-line legislation. The NBAC recommended that Congress pass a law forbidding reproductive SCNT with a five-year sunset provision and a number of European nations, including the United Kingdom, proscribe reproductive SCNT.

A narrow anticloning law, especially one with a sunset provision, would have certain merits. It would reflect the sentiments of many, if public opinion polls, media commentary, and interest group statements are guides. If narrowly drawn, it would avoid charges of being overbroad or vague and it would arguably not detract from reproductive liberty, especially when safety questions remain and many alternative ways of conceiving genetically related children are available. A circumscribed law barring this one act would add the voice of the United States to a fairly universal sentiment against reproductive SCNT.

On the other hand, a law targeting a single reproductive technique would set an unusual precedent. This would be the first time the government would make criminal a medical technique, and a hypothetical one at that. The usual way of discouraging research in biotechnology is to withhold federal funds; other technologies posing concerns, such as r-DNA technology, were slowed by means other than legislative bans. An anticloning law might set precedent for looking to Congress when other ethically questionable technologies arise, making Congress a court of first rather than last resort. Moreover, the bar for enacting a law would be set low because the injuries of reproductive SCNT have not been carefully articulated beyond safety, and even here the matter is unresolved (*Washington Fax* 2001b).

Another problem with legislation is that passing a law will not end the matter. It might forbid one narrow activity, but it would still be undermined by technological changes. Technique-based laws tend to be brittle, a "crude tool" (Berg and Singer 1998). They are too often underinclusive (not covering what is intended) or overinclusive (covering more than intended) (Knoppers 1997, G4–G6). For example, if it could be determined how to mix the somatic cell nuclei of two people in one egg, would this be forbidden under an anticloning law (Solter and Gearhart 1999, 1470)? It is difficult to know how technologies will develop, and unexpected developments can turn technique-specific laws into pronouncements of limited utility at best and relics at worst. Even as carefully constructed an embryo research law as that in the United Kingdom had to be revisited because its framers anticipated several kinds of cloning but not reproductive SCNT.

Legislation with a Broad Arc

In 2001, the House voted to approve a bill, H.R. 2505, that would forbid all human SCNT technology (U.S. House 2001c). The purpose of this and similar bills is to prevent the temptation to use SCNT for reproduction. If scientists gain skills and knowledge from SCNT research, the argument goes, it is inevitable that someone will transfer an embryo created through SCNT to a woman's uterus. The likelihood will increase further if couples request the technique and if some researchers are motivated by the desire to be first in human cloning. The answer, with this policy approach, is to prevent competency from developing by barring all human SCNT technology.

In late 2001, investigators at Advanced Cell Technology announced they had created early-stage human embryos through SCNT as a step toward eventual therapy (Cibelli et al. 2001). They unsuccessfully transferred from human skin cells to eleven enucleated eggs. When they transferred nuclei from human cumulus cells to four enucleated eggs, however, they found that one egg cleaved to six cells and two cleaved to four cells before ceasing to divide. Under a bill such as H.R. 2505, this research would be illegal. Some variants of legislation with a broad arc would go further, such as laws in California and Louisiana that bar all human nuclear transfer from egg, embryo, fetal somatic cells, and adult somatic cells.

Serious problems attend this approach. It would be difficult if not impossible to craft an anti-SCNT law that would not take a wide swath of protected activity with it as researchers sought to steer clear of the proscribed activity. Moreover, justifying the broad arc would present challenges because of the speculative nature of the injuries. While one could conceivably justify barring embryo transfer on the grounds of risk to mother and potential child (as extrapolated from animal studies), on what grounds would one justify barring all SCNT technology? The proffered reason—to prevent a dangerous activity down the road—is amorphous and logically flawed. If this is justified as a way of saving embryos, that too would fail to withstand scrutiny because embryos are not persons under the law. Moreover, embryos are lost in many aspects of research and practice; to bar this one use would impose a dubious distinction.

Barring all SCNT would raise the possibility of barring science because policymakers do not like the science, which hardly respects the vitality of the scientific endeavor and which would pose an unfortunate precedent. It would also quash research that may never lead to reproductive uses, such as therapeutic SCNT or other uses not yet imagined. Moreover, this intrusive prior restraint would be for naught because it would not stop the practice. Policymakers in numerous nations are grappling with the issue and not all will enact restrictive legislation or go further than denying funding for the research.

If the world's largest biotechnology producer, the United States, bows out of SCNT technology altogether by making it illegal, the nation has denied itself a leadership role in policy development. Irrespective of the question of competitiveness on the market is the separate matter of policy innovation. The United States can lead by example and procedure most effectively if it is a player. This does not mean that its scientists need to practice SCNT to be involved; it does mean, however, that by preemptively barring all human SCNT technology the country will absent itself from effective policy initiatives and development.

Existing Regulatory Mechanisms

As discussed in previous chapters, the existing regulatory apparatus includes FDA oversight, tort law for policing negligence, the *Fertility Clinic Success Rate and Certification Act of 1992*, judicial interpetations, laws in states where opinion is especially intense, and self-monitoring by involved professions and corporations. This approach places trust in the existing system, and it may or may not be accompanied by the conviction that reproductive cloning is a serious threat to society. People who lean toward this approach may not resist adjustments to it, but they basically believe the apparatus is supple enough to accommodate whatever challenges reproductive SCNT poses.

In support of this approach, one can point to the successful practice of biotechnology in the United States where interests in economic development have been balanced with protections for public health and welfare. While many questions remain about r-DNA technology in crops, the introduction of the technology thus far has been gradual and free from environmental disasters. Despite abundant concerns about the safety of IVF and its variants, children conceived through ART have no more serious birth disorders than children conceived without intervention, and ICRI, preimplantation genetic diagnosis, and other innovations have proceeded without obvious incident. In fact, owing to governmental avoidance of ART issues, the practice has developed with the most minimal use of governmental resources. Another merit of the status quo model is that it is pluralistic, with numerous places for adjustments. It does not have a congressional centerpiece, but it admits democratic involvement through case law, which invites friends of the court briefs and public attention; tort outcomes, which can draw negative publicity and incentives for self-policing; public notices from the FDA; and lobbying activities of professional associations, patient advocacy groups, and the biotechnology industry.

This approach falters, however, in that it insufficiently acknowledges public reservations about reproductive SCNT. In addition, it eschews the opportunity to build a creative policy framework that will set the stage for future problematic technologies.

Adjustments to Existing Regulatory Mechanisms

Adjusting the existing regulatory apparatus has merits and drawbacks similar to those raised by the previous approach. A broad category, it varies depending on the intent and nature of the proposed changes. For example, amending the *Food, Drug, and Cosmetic Act* to reinforce the FDA's authority in overseeing reproductive SCNT would be a significant regulatory adjustment. Establishing a deliberative body to discuss the implications of reproductive and genetic technologies would have fewer regulatory implications because added discussions, in their ability to clarify issues, may forestall decision making. The early years of reproductive cloning policy suggest four types of adjustments, as identified below.

Science Oversight

What stands out in the existing regulatory apparatus is the near total absence of scientific oversight by the federal government for reproductive technologies, as discussed in chapter 7. If ARTs and genetic technologies such as preimplantation genetic diagnosis have developed safely, they have done so with a measure of luck given the shifting of the experimental setting from the laboratory to clinical practice. The missing federal hand is especially ironic because it relates to reproductive issues that are highly salient to many.

Research funding invites federal science oversight. A double-edged policy that enables research but brings restrictions with it, funding opens scientific inquiry to the public, requires peer review to ensure high-quality research, and provides the resources for sustained research. Since the government is not going to fund reproductive SCNT, the federal voice for reproductive and genetic technologies must be coached gradually and indirectly. One way of doing this is to expand the range of studies subject to purview by the RAC or establish a new RAC-like body. A logical starting place, as several policy commentators have recommended, is to empower the RAC to review research involving IGMs (Palmer and Cook-Deegan in press; Frankel and Chapman 2000; 2001; Parens and Juengst 2001).

The RAC has never reviewed IGM proposals. As stated in its Appendix M:

> The RAC and its Subcommittee will not at present entertain proposals for germ line alterations . . . in germ line alterations, a specific attempt is made to introduce genetic changes into the germ (reproductive) cells of an individual, with the aim of changing the set of genes passed on to the individual's offspring (NIH 1990).

Consequently, the RAC could be empowered to review IGM protocols and issues by changing Appendix M and by broadly defining IGMs to include egg cell nuclear transfer, ooplasm transfer, and other techniques that go beyond the above definition of splicing of nuclear DNA. Egg cell nuclear transfer, done to circumvent mitochondrial disease or enable older women to conceive, would be an IGM because the resulting child would inherit the nuclear DNA of the mother and the mitochondrial DNA of the egg donor (Bonnicksen 1998). Although not cloning, this technology would open RAC review to a limited (noncloning) form of nuclear transfer. Presumably, reproductive SCNT would also be an IGM if a person's somatic cell nucleus were transferred to a donor's enucleated egg and the resulting child inherited the donor's mitochondrial DNA.

As envisioned by Palmer and Cook-Deegan (in press), expanded oversight by the RAC or a RAC-like body would have several components. Among other things, the overseeing body would (1) review all IGM protocols, whether privately or publicly funded; (2) follow IRB review; (3) be located outside the NIH to avoid conflicts of interest when the NIH is the funding agency; and (4) initiate review only when "substantive" ethical issues arise and not simply automatically when an IGM technique is present.

RAC oversight has the merit of inviting public review by a body with a reputation for rigorous review of gene therapy protocols. This would be a national-level process involving scientific review by experts who are not necessarily available at the local level. The RAC could undertake these new responsibilities only with expanded financial resources.

The purpose of this adjustment would be to activate an existing, well-regarded policy mechanism for technologies on the horizon. In a sign of a gradual movement in this direction, the RAC has held two gene therapy conferences to discuss the possibility that somatic cell gene therapy might inadvertently alter germ cells. In the first, held in 1999 and discussed in chapter 7, RAC members discussed the possibility that in utero gene therapy on fetuses might inadvertently modify the fetus's germ cells. In the second, held in December 2001, the RAC set the stage for an open discussion of issues raised by a study put on hold by the FDA. In this study, investigators found traces of DNA from the vector used in a somatic cell gene therapy study in the semen of a volunteer research subject (Marshall 2001). While the meeting yielded no clear conclusions, it provided an open forum for the airing of ethical and scientific concerns. It also demonstrated the RAC's utility as a forum for discussing germ-line issues.

Enlarging the RAC's mission to review genetic modifications and expanding the definition of germ-line therapy to include inheritable mitochondrial interventions would put the RAC in a position to review issues related to nuclear transfer. RAC review could be minimal (review ethical issues and develop guidelines), moderate (review IGM protocols submitted for funding if funding for IGMs has been authorized), or extensive (reviewing all protocols, private and public).

Just as it makes sense to use the RAC as a policy vehicle for reviewing ethical issues and developing guidelines, so does it make sense to use IGMs as a scientific vehicle for including research related to reproductive SCNT. For one thing, one or more forms of nuclear transfer may facilitate IGMs, as they did in the case of Polly the transgenic lamb. This foretells an eventual intersection between nuclear transfer and IGMs for therapeutic use. For another thing, government funding of IGMs is not an excessively remote prospect. On the contrary, IGMs have a narrow but growing support (see, e.g., Stock and Campbell 2000; Munson and Davis 1992; Zimmerman 1991). In contrast to reproductive SCNT, which is of doubtful need, IGMs can be framed as offering a valid medical intervention. Ironically, this perceived need may well come from individuals who seek to protect human embryos. A case can be built for IGMs if they prevent the birth of children with serious diseases or conditions through a positive intervention (modifying the embryo or gametes) rather than a negative intervention (using preimplantation genetic diagnosis, discarding affected embryos, and selectively transferring only unaffected embryos). One might well see a phenomenon similar to that arising with ES cell research, where persons opposed to abortion favored ES cell research because of the benefits that might arise. With IGMs, persons opposed to abortion and embryo research might not only support IGMs but also feel an obligation to pursue an alternative to embryo destruction. In any case, IGMs may be poised as stepping-off points for federal deliberations about reproductive and genetic technologies.

Product and Process

Another adjustment is to strengthen the FDA's jurisdiction over reproductive SCNT. One approach is to amend its authorizing statutes, but a technique-based amendment would have infirmities similar to those raised by technique-based anticloning laws. A more flexible alternative is to rely on FDA discretion to expand its range of oversight through policy statements and guidance documents, as it did with somatic cell and gene therapies in the 1990s. In anticipation of this possibility, a wider discussion among policymakers is advisable to clarify on what grounds risk analysis will proceed.

An issue that has divided policymakers in the matter of agricultural biotechnology is whether genetically modified foodstuffs should be regulated on the basis of the process by which they are created (r-DNA technology) or on the basis of the safety of the end product (foods). Posed another way, there are differences of opinion of whether regulation should focus on the "genetic technique or on the characteristics of the resulting product" (Miller 1997, 2). Agricultural policy after the onset of r-DNA technology followed a cautious approach in which the mere presence of the technology prompted extra safeguards. At first, no field trials of r-DNA crops were allowed, then the studies started on a case-by-case basis with RAC review, and then RAC oversight was lifted. This policy history was unique to r-DNA research and was triggered by the technology itself (Miller 1997, 138). In the late 1980s the National Academy of Sciences issued a report endorsing the product-based approach for biotechnology (Miller 1997, 9) and the FDA follows it in its many areas of regulation. For the most part, a product-based approach prevails in the United States, where the properties of the product, such as genetically modified corn, capture the attention of regulators. In Europe, in contrast, public sympathy leans toward a precautionary principle in which

r-DNA technology prompts heightened oversight. The precautionary principle recognizes incomplete knowledge and cautions that one
should not proceed in the presence of risk even if that risk has not
been empirically demonstrated (NCB 1999, 8).

The product/process distinction arises in legislative debates over
reproductive SCNT because bills that would outlaw all SCNT technology are process-based proposals. These bills target SCNT as dangerous, not because of physical risks but because of its status as a supposed marker in the path to reproductive SCNT. The process-based
approach is clearly evident in California and Louisiana, which barred
all forms of nuclear transfer, including egg cell nuclear transfer and
other forms unrelated to cloning. Missing from the debates is a serious consideration of whether all forms of nuclear transfer should be
indicted and, if so, why.

Arguably, the FDA is, in effect, although not in intent, straddling a
process-based as well as product-based approach in matters relating to
nuclear transfer. In his letter to IRB chairs in 1998, Stuart Nightingale, associate commissioner for health affairs, reminded investigators
they must submit an IND to the FDA before proceeding with clinical
studies using "cloning technology" (Nightingale 1998). This letter
came after news stories indicated that some researchers were considering egg cell nuclear transfer. Its timing seemed to equate egg cell nuclear transfer with a cloning technology simply because it relied on
nuclear transfer. In a letter in 2001 to unnamed researchers, the FDA
again included egg cell nuclear transfer as an example of a technique
over which the FDA had jurisdiction (Zoon 2001).

Product-based reasoning figured in these letters inasmuch as a manipulated embryo could be regarded as an unsafe product that should
not, under today's incomplete understanding, be transferred to a
woman's uterus. Yet the reasoning is unclear, which illustrates the ad-
visability of policy deliberations to explore and clarify principles of
oversight. This does not promise to be an easy task. As Martha
Carter points out, the new techniques *are* more process than product,
thereby blurring the lines between prevailing concepts (Carter 1996,
379).

The task is to decide how risk-based analysis should proceed for
reproductive SCNT and other forms of nuclear transfer. Should nuclear transfer in itself trigger heightened oversight? If yes, why and
how? When in early testimony before the NBAC, John Robertson

and Ruth Macklin asked those who wanted to ban cloning to produce evidence of concrete harms from reproductive SCNT, they in effect were arguing against a process-based approach in which the presence of SCNT would in itself trigger restrictions (NBAC 1997b). A product-based orientation would posit that the government should step in only if tangible harms were posed to the child, family, or society. With a process-based orientation, however, all procedures involving nuclear transfer would trigger review.

Deliberative Forum

How best can new technologies be discussed and debated? Now that the NBAC has expired, what will be the U.S. equivalent of the NCB or the HGC in the United Kingdom? Where might a "trustworthy, neutral source of expertise on emerging issues," a body where diverse people publicly examine technologies as they emerge and think prospectively about managing innovation, be located (Malakoff 2001, 2230)?

One possibility is to establish by Executive Order a body similar to the NBAC. President Clinton had done this with the NBAC, giving it an initial tenure of two years and then extending it until 2001. According to the NBAC's charter, the commission's first priority was to examine ways to protect participants in human research (NIH, Office of Science and Technology 1996, 1). It was authorized to conduct hearings, solicit information, and contract for background papers. Departments and agencies were asked to cooperate with NBAC requests for information. The NBAC was to hold ten or more public meetings a year, with advance notice in the *Federal Register*. Members were solicited through an open nomination process.

President Bush performed a similar action when he set up the PCB by Executive Order in late 2001 (President, Executive Order 2001). Headed by Leon Kass from the University of Chicago, the PCB was to have up to eighteen members appointed by the president for two-year terms and from different fields. Its mission was broadly to (1) advise the president on bioethical issues, (2) provide a forum for the discussion of bioethical issues, and (3) explore opportunities for international collaboration (President, Executive Order 2001, 59851). In support of this mission it was expected that the PCB would provide a context for airing diverse views and not necessarily achieving consensus.

Creating a body through Executive Order can be done efficiently and without entering the congressional arena, which is predictably roiled by bioethical issues. This approach can yield useful insights in a short period of time. On the other hand, a body established in the executive branch is susceptible to appointments reflecting the ideology of the president. In addition, it does not have the status of a body created by Congress.

During the NBAC cloning hearings, for example, one witness told of the ending of the EAB, which had been created in the DHEW. The EAB had such limited visibility that legislators stopped funding it because they did not know its functions (NBAC 1999b, 2). When appropriating funds for a commission to study the protection of human research subjects, some members of Congress wondered why both the commission and the EAB were needed. A staff member at DHEW, who served as a last-minute substitute witness, did not know why the two boards were needed. Hearing no justification for funding two boards and not knowing the EAB's function, Congress withdrew its funding for the EAB.

Although using Congress to set up an NBAC-like body has appeal, history shows that Congress has been less than successful, as seen by its failed attempt to staff the bipartisan Biomedical Ethics Board in 1985. In addition, establishing bodies to explore new technologies is not a salient issue in Congress, as indicated by its dismemberment in 1985 of the Office of Technology Assessment (OTA), a science advisory body that developed policy reports on such issues as genetic discrimination and infertility treatment (Malakoff 2001, 2229). In the shadow of an administration slow to appoint scientific advisors, members of Congress display little enthusiasm about establishing a new science advisory body. As one reporter said of suggestions in 2001 to establish an OTA equivalent, "convincing Congress it needs a new OTA will be about as easy as cloning a dinosaur" (Malakoff 2001, 2230). This is not to negate efforts to establish a forum; it is to warn of the difficulties of doing so.

Preemptive Thinking

What will happen if reproductive SCNT enters the world of procreative medicine earlier than expected and despite precautions? How much effort should go into preemptively thinking about policy in the event reproductive SCNT is one day practiced? Presumably, resistance to reproductive SCNT will not be unassailable or permanent. Not only will safety issues be addressed, but one may expect a softening of attitudes as has occurred with other technologies after the initial shock subsides. Already observers are questioning the assumption that reproductive SCNT will necessarily be harmful, and the ready list of clients for the Raelians (Clonaid) points to a germinating client demand. Technological optimism is also coming to the fore, as is general curiosity, articulated by Richard Dawkins, who asks, "Mightn't you, in your heart of hearts, quite like to be cloned?" He goes on to say,

> I find it a personally riveting thought that I could watch a small copy of myself, fifty years younger and wearing a baseball hat instead of a British Empire pith helmet, nurtured through the early decades of the twenty-first century. Mightn't it feel almost like turning back your personal clock fifty years? And mightn't it be wonderful to advise your junior copy on where you went wrong, and how to do it better? Isn't this, in (sometimes sadly) watered-down form, one of the motives that drives people to breed children in the ordinary way, by sexual reproduction? (Dawkins 1998, 55).

One can also see a gradual entry of cloning into everyday culture, as with Genetic Savings and Clone, a company formed to store cells from pets for cloning, and a gift of $2 million to Texas A & M University to clone a family dog Missy (Talbot 2000, 21). These seemingly innocuous potential uses of animal cloning, writes Margaret Talbot "[make] human cloning not just more technically plausible, but more emotionally plausible" (Talbot 2000, 22).

As acclimation sets in, the arguments that were once taken at face value look less persuasive under careful scrutiny. For example, a worst-case scenario for reproductive cloning typically has the resulting child burdened by expectations that he or she will be like the donor. Yet a worst-case scenario could also be visualized for gamete or embryo donation, where the child's genetic forebears often remain anonymous (Bonnicksen 2001a). It is not immediately clear why a child who shares a genome with one parent in reproductive SCNT and who perhaps knows too much about her genes is more harmed than a child born from gamete or embryo donation who may know too little of his genetic heritage. Nor is it immediately evident why reducing the participants to one genome donor in reproductive SCNT would be more problematic than expanding the parties to conception in donation arrangements, with the subsequent potential for protracted custody conflicts.

Although the popular literature is replete with fantastic scenarios, little discussion ensues about how reproductive SCNT realistically might unfold in the clinical setting. Assume, for example, that a couple with dual infertility (he has immotile sperm and she has no ovaries) visit a clinic. The couple wonders why they should turn to anonymous donors when they could use one of their genomes to produce a child through reproductive SCNT. Assume in a second example that a couple with dual infertility feels uncomfortable using the genome of one of them but they have a good friend who has agreed to be the somatic cell donor. The friend is flattered; she would enjoy watching a young girl with her genome raised by her good friends. All the details are worked out, say the couple. Why should they use anonymous donors when they can use the genome of a known friend? Assume in a third example that a single fertile man, age fifty-two, requests that his somatic cells be used to initiate a pregnancy with a surrogate who, after the birth, will relinquish parental rights to him. If he can legally impregnate a woman, he argues, why should he not be able to use his body cells to produce offspring? The difference between reproductive SCNT and ordinary conception is, he says, a matter of degree.

In the absence of a ban on reproductive SCNT, decision making shifts to the clinical sector, where clinicians make judgments about when to proceed and under what circumstances. At present, various professional bodies have called for a moratorium on reproductive SCNT and for further discussions about its implications (Ethics Committee of the ASRM 2000). In the event of changing conditions, however, the clinician may have no ready response to such requests, as illustrated above. If demonstrated to be safe for animals, which is not in the forecast at present, should reproductive SCNT be gradually introduced into the clinical setting? What, if any, preemptive steps might be taken to prepare for that eventuality?

The danger of engaging in clinically oriented ethical inquiry is that it might be interpreted to mean that reproductive SCNT is regarded as acceptable and/or inevitable. Yet anticipatory deliberations do not necessarily endorse reproductive cloning or accept its inevitability.

On the contrary, such deliberations can add rigor to ethical argumentation. Limits on cloning will have greater staying power if distinctions, rationales, and guiding principles for clinical use are proposed and defended. On the other hand, if the technology is never used with humans, such anticipatory discussions can illuminate discussions about other contentious techniques that may yet unfold. The bottom line is that many issues remain to be explored, and policy exists on all levels, including informal policies developed in the clinical setting where clinicians develop rules about who to admit, what procedures to offer, how fast to proceed, and what limits will be placed on services offered. These policies are basic building blocks of ART policy, yet their potential for informing the broader policy debate is not always appreciated.

The role played by the medical community would be most important in the developmental stages, when working standards are developed that can be amended more easily than legislation. Anticipatory guidelines can also set the stage for future regulation, either by substituting for it or by presenting a model on which laws may be crafted. Regulating nearer to the fact of reproductive SCNT is consistent with responses to other medical innovations. It enables a policy based on observation rather than speculation and it can avoid the errors that arise when policymakers in one decade presume that they can anticipate the state of science in the next.

A CHANGING METAPHOR

A prevailing metaphor in reproductive SCNT places us, analogously speaking, on a San Francisco cable car inching its way up a steep hill, click by click, where the top is visible but riders can only guess what lies on the other side of the crest. An alternative metaphor replaces the cable car with the more pedestrian Amtrak train lumbering across the Illinois plains on its journey from Chicago to New Orleans. The journey yields no nail-biting grades or fog-enshrouded landmarks. Instead, riders experience little more than occasional lurches and stops and a landscape of unremarkable silos and roads that head straight east or straight west. This metaphor places us not on the ascent to a blind crest but instead on a flat plain, in the middle of a journey, with undistinguished features. The few surprises in this train journey do not overpower the massive steel engine that pulls its cargo along, competently if not colorfully. Exchanging the San Francisco cable car for a midwest Amtrak train means taking stock of what reasonably may be done to manage developments on the pike.

There is danger in adopting a less-spectacular metaphor of reproductive cloning and in challenging the sense that dramatic landmarks are upon us requiring bold and speedy responses. Yet there is danger too in adding to what can be a conceit that our issues are the most vivid and our technologies are the most threatening to humankind. Future policy in the area of innovative reproductive technologies will likely be incremental and cautious. Given that the political system is internally wired for cautious change, this is hardly surprising. An approach that adjusts the existing regulatory framework conforms with the incremental nature of science and the political system. The train is, indeed, out of the station, and the conductor's resources for creative policy are considerable.

REFERENCES

Aker, Janet. 2001. "Stem Cell Researchers, Patient Advocates Intervene in Suit to Halt Federal Funding of Embryonic Stem Cell Research." *Washington Fax*, 21 May, 1–2.

Aldous, Peter. 1990. "Pro-Life Actions Backfire." *Nature* 345, no. 6270: 7.

American Association for the Advancement of Science/Institute for Civil Society. 1999. *Stem Cell Research and Applications: Monitoring the Frontiers of Biomedical Research.* Washington, DC: American Association for the Advancement of Science. Available at: www.aaas.org/spp/dspp/sfrl/projects/stem/main.htm.

American College of Obstetricians and Gynecologists. Committee on Ethics. 1994. "Committee Opinion on Preembryo Research." Washington, DC: American College of Obstetricians and Gynecologists.

American Society for Reproductive Medicine. 1999. "CDC Releases ART Lab Standards." *ASRM Bulletin* 1, no. 11: 1.

———. 2001. "FDA Releases Part 3 of Proposed Rule for Reproductive Tissue." *ASRM Bulletin* 3, no. 2: 1.

Anderson, G. B. 1999. "Embryonic Stem Cells in Agricultural Species." In *Transgenic Animals in Agriculture*, edited by J. D. Murray, G. B. Anderson, A. M. Oberbauer, and M. M. McGloughlin, 1–18. New York: CABI Publishing.

Andrews, Lori B. 1997. "The Current and Future Legal Status of Cloning." In *Cloning Human Beings: Report and Recommendations of the National Bioethics Advisory Commission, Volume II: Commissioned Papers*, F1–F90. Rockville, MD: National Bioethics Advisory Commission.

———. 1999. *The Clone Age: Adventures in the New World of Reproductive Technology.* New York: Henry Holt.

———. 2000. "State Regulation of Embryo Stem Cell Research." In *Ethical Issues in Human Stem Cell Research, Volume II: Commissioned Papers*, by National Bioethics Advisory Commission, A1–A13. Rockville, MD: National Bioethics Advisory Commission.

Angergame, Lisa, and Jane S. Tierney. 1996. "California Enacts 'Fertility Fraud' Laws." *Fertility News* 30, no. 4: 24.

Annas, George J. 1998a. "The Shadowlands—Secrets, Lies, and Assisted Reproduction." *New England Journal of Medicine* 339, no. 13: 935–39.

Annas, George J., Arthur Caplan, and Sherman Elias. 1996. "The Politics of Human-Embryo Research—Avoiding Ethical Gridlock." *New England Journal of Medicine* 334, no. 20: 1329–32.

Australian Academy of Science. 1999. *On Human Cloning: A Position Statement.* Canberra: Australian Academy of Science, 4 February.

———. 2001. *Human Stem Cell Research.* Canberra: Australian Academy of Science, 18 April.

Australian Health Ethics Council. 1998. "Report on Scientific, Ethical and Regulatory Considerations Relevant to Cloning of Human Beings." Canberra: National Health and Medical Research Council, Australian Health Ethics Council, December.

Bahadur, G. 2001. "The Human Rights Act (1998) and Its Impact on Reproductive Tissues." *Human Reproduction* 16, no. 4: 785–89.

Beach, Judith E. 1999. "The New RAC: Restructuring of the National Institutes of Health Recombinant DNA Advisory Committee." *Food and Drug Law Journal* 54, no. 1: 49–53.

Berg, Paul, and Maxine Singer. 1998. "Regulating Human Cloning." *Science* 282: 413.

Biotechnology Industry Organization. 1999. "Oversight of Gene Therapy: A Position Paper." Washington, DC: Biotechnology Industry Organization, 7 December.

Bonnicksen, Andrea L. 1989. *In Vitro Fertilization: Building Policy from Laboratories to Legislatures*. New York: Columbia University Press.

———. 1997. "Procreation by Cloning: Crafting Anticipatory Guidelines." *Journal of Law, Medicine and Ethics* 25: 273–82.

———. 1998. "Transplanting Nuclei between Human Eggs: Implications for Germ-Line Genetics." *Politics and the Life Sciences* 17, no. 1: 3–10.

———. 2001a. "Human Reproductive Cloning: Thinking About Clinic-Based Ethics." *Fertility and Sterility* 75, no. 6: 1057–58.

———. 2001b. "Human Embryonic Stem Cell Research: The Role of Private Policy." In *Reproductive Medicine in the Twenty-First Century: Proceedings of the Seventeenth World Congress on Fertility and Sterility, Melbourne, Australia*. Edited by D. L. Healy, G. T. Kovacs, R. McLachlan, and O. Rodriguez-Armas, 21–29. London: Parthenon Publishing Group.

Brody, Baruch A. 1998. *The Ethics of Biomedical Research: An International Perspective*. New York: Oxford University Press.

———. 2000. "Human Subjects Research, Law, FDA Rules." In *Encyclopedia of Ethical, Legal, and Policy Issues in Biotechnology*, edited by Thomas J. Murray and Maxwell J. Mehlman, 675–81. New York: John Wiley & Sons.

Brownback, Sam, Don Nickles, Jon Kyl, Bob Smith, Jesse Helms, Michael B. Enzi, and John Ashcroft, U.S. Senate. 1999. Letter to Donna E. Shalala, Secretary of Health and Human Services, 12 February. Photocopy. Andrea Bonnicksen, private collection, DeKalb, IL.

Bruni, Frank. 2001. "Unexpected Priority: Stem Cell Research's Rise as a Test for Bush." *New York Times*, 14 July, A10.

Buckingham, Margaret. 2000. "A Cellular Cornucopia." *Nature* 408: 773.

Butler, Declan. 1998. "Patent Clash Looming Over Cloning Techniques?" *Nature* 394: 409.

Byk, J. C. 1994. "Bioethics within the Council of Europe: The Protection of Genetic Information." In *Bioethics for the People by the People*, edited by D. R. J. Macer, 68–73. Christchurch, New Zealand: Eubois Ethics Institute.

Callahan, Daniel. 1990. *What Kind of Life? The Limits of Medical Progress*. New York: Touchstone.

———. 2000. "Death and the Research Imperative." *New England Journal of Medicine* 342, no. 9: 654–56.

Canada. 1997. "Bill C-247, An Act to Amend the Criminal Code." 36th Parliament, 1st sess., 46 Elizabeth II. Available at: www.parl.gc.ca/36/1/parlbus/chambu. Accessed 1 March 1998.

Canada. Royal Commission on New Reproductive Technologies. 1993. *Proceed with Care: Final Report of the Royal Commission on New Reproductive Technologies*. Ottawa: Minister of Government Services Canada.

Canadian Institutes of Health Research. 2001a. "About the CIHR." Available at: cihr.ca/about-cihr/who_we_are/fold_e.html. Accessed on 8 February 2001.

———. 2001b. *Human Stem Cell Research: Opportunities for Health and Ethical Perspectives: A Discussion Paper*. Ottawa: Canadian Institutes of Health Research.

———. 2001c. "Human Stem Cell Research: Opportunities for Health and Ethical Perspectives. Request for Feedback." Available at: www.cihr.ca/news/forums/ stem_cell/issues. Accessed on 19 April 2001.

Carmen, Ira H. 1985. *Cloning and the Constitution: An Inquiry into Governmental Policy-making and Genetic Experimentation*. Madison: University of Wisconsin Press.

———. 1997. "Should Human Cloning Be Criminalized?" *Journal of Law and Politics* 13, no. 4: 745–58.

Carter, Martha J. 1996. "The Ability of Current Biologics Law to Accommodate Emerging Technologies." *Food and Drug Law Journal* 51, no. 3: 375–80.

Center for Bioethics and Human Dignity. 1999. "On Human Embryos and Stem Cell Research: An Appeal for Legally and Ethically Responsible Science and Public Policy." Available at www.stemcellresearch.org/statement.htm. Accessed on 21 November 1999.

Chan, A. W. S., T. Dominko, C. M. Luetjens, E. Neuber, C. Martinovich, L. Hewitson, C. R. Simerly, G. P. Schatten. 2000. "Clonal Propagation of Primate Offspring by Embryo Splitting." *Science* 287: 317–19.

Cibelli, Jose B., Ann A. Kiessling, Kerrianne Cunniff, Charlotte Richards, Robert P. Laza, and Michael D. West. 2001. "Somatic Cell Nuclear Transfer in Humans: Pronuclear and Early Embryonic Development." *E-biomed: The Journal of Regenerative Medicine* 2 (26 November): 25–31.

Clinton, William, President of the United States. 1997a. Letter to Harold Shapiro, Chair of National Bioethics Advisory Commission, 24 February. Reprinted in *Cloning Human Beings: Report and Recommendations of the National Bioethics Advisory Commission*, by National Bioethics Commission. Rockville, MD: National Bioethics Advisory Commission.

———. 1997b. "Remarks by President on Cloning." The White House, Office of the Press Secretary, 4 March. Washington, DC. E-mail hard copy. Andrea Bonnicksen, private collection, DeKalb, IL.

———. 1998. Letter to Harold Shapiro, chair of National Bioethics Advisory Commission, 14 November. Photocopy. Andrea Bonnicksen, private collection, DeKalb, IL.

Clinton, William, and Albert Gore. 1997. "Remarks By President Bill Clinton and VP Al Gore at the Presentation of the National Bioethics Advisory Commission Report on Cloning." White House Briefing, 9 June. Available at: web.lexis-nexis.com/ congcomp. Accessed on 5 November 1999.

Cohen, Cynthia B. 1997. "Unmanaged Care: The Need to Regulate New Reproductive Technologies in the United States." *Bioethics Forum* 3/4: 348–65.

Cohen, I. Glenn. 2000. "Administrative Developments: New Human Subjects Research Guidelines for IRBs." *Journal of Law, Medicine and Ethics* 28, no. 3: 305–07.

Cohen, Susan. 1997. "What Is a Baby? Inside America's Unresolved Debate about the Ethics of Cloning." *Washington Post Magazine*, 12 October, 12–17, 24–29.

Congressional Record. 1997–2000. Washington, DC.

Council of Europe. 1998. "Additional Protocol to the Convention for the Protection of Human Rights and Dignity of the Human Being with regard to the Application of Biology and Medicine, on the Prohibition of Cloning Human Beings." ETS No. 168. Additional Protocol to the ETS No. 164. Paris, 12.I.1998. Available at: www.coe.fr/eng/legaltxt/168e.htm. Accessed on 1 February 1998.

Council for Responsible Genetics. 1997. "Position Statement on Cloning." Cambridge, MA: Council for Responsible Genetics, 11 March.

Crockin, Susan L. 2001. "Legally Speaking." *ASRM News* 35, no. 1: 9–10.

Dawkins, Richard. 1998. "What's Wrong with Cloning?" In *Clones and Clones: Facts and Fantasies about Human Cloning*, edited by Martha C. Nussbaum and Cass R. Sunstein, 54–66. New York: Norton.

"Declaration of Helsinki." 1995. In *Encyclopedia of Bioethics*, rev. ed., edited by Warren Thomas Reich, 5:2765–67. New York: Macmillan; London: Prentice Hall International.

Delgado, Richard, and David R. Miller. 1978. "God, Galileo, and Government: Toward Constitutional Protection for Scientific Inquiry." *Washington Law Review* 53: 349–404.

The Detroit News. 1998. "State Senate Bans Human Cloning." 29 April. Available at: detnews.com/1998/metro. Accessed on 16 February 2001.

Dickey, Jay, Henry J. Hyde, Joe Barton, Duncan Hunter, Spencer Bachus, Ron Packard, Dan Burton, W. J. (Billy) Tauzin, and others, U.S. House. 1999. Letter to Donna E. Shalala, Secretary of Health and Human Services, 11 February. Andrea Bonnicksen, private collection, DeKalb, IL.

Dickson, David. 2000. "European Panel Rejects Creation of Human Embryos for Research." *Nature* 408: 277.

———. 2001. "Parliament Gives Green Light to Stem-Cell Research." *Nature* 409: 5.

Doerflinger, Richard M. 1999. "The Ethics of Funding Embryonic Stem Cell Research: A Catholic Viewpoint." *Kennedy Institute of Ethics Journal* 9, no. 2: 137–50.

Dommel, F. W., Jr., and D. Alexander. 1997. "The Convention on Human Rights and Biomedicine of the Council of Europe." *Kennedy Institute of Ethics Journal* 7, no. 3: 259–76.

Dorff, Elliott, Nancy J. Duff, Margaret Farley, and Abdulaziz Sachedina. 1999. Letter to J. Dennis Hastert, U.S. House, 12 October. Andrea Bonnicksen, private collection, DeKalb, IL.

Dworkin, Roger B. 1996. *Limits: The Role of the Law in Bioethical Decision Making*. Bloomington: Indiana University Press.

Eisenberg, Leon. 1999. "Would Cloned Humans Really Be Like Sheep?" *New England Journal of Medicine* 340, no. 6: 471–75.

Eiseman, Elisa. 1997. "Views of Scientific Societies and Professional Associations on Human Nuclear Transfer Cloning Research. In *Cloning Human Beings: Report and Recommendations of the National Bioethics Advisory Commission, Volume II: Commissioned Papers*, C1–C31. Rockville, MD: National Bioethics Advisory Commission.

———. 2000. "Cloning, Policy Issues." In *Encyclopedia of Ethical, Legal, and Policy Issues in Biotechnology*, edited by Thomas J. Murray and Maxwell J. Mehlman, 157–72. New York: John Wiley & Sons.

Eisenstadt v. Baird, 405 US 438 (1972).

Environment News Service. 2001. "UK Legalizes Cloning of Human Embryos." Available at: ens.lycos.com/ens/jan2001. Accessed on 30 March 2001.

Ethics Committee of the American Society for Reproductive Medicine. 2000. "Human Somatic Cell Nuclear Transfer (Cloning)." *Fertility and Sterility* 74, no. 5: 873–76.

European Commission. 1997. "Communiqué Adopted by the Summit of the Eight." Twenty-third Western Economic Summit. Bulletin EU, 7/8-1997. Available at: europa.eu.int/abc/doc/off/bull/en/9707/p000519.htm. Accessed on 8 June 1998.

European Commission. European Group on Ethics in Science and New Technologies. 1999. "Report to the European Commission: Ethical Aspects of Research Involving the Use of Human Embryos in the Context of the Fifth Framework Program (November 23, 1998)." *Politics and the Life Sciences* 18, no. 1: 123–29.

———. 2000. "Ethical Aspects of Human Stem Cell Research and Use." Opinion no. 15, 14 November. Available at: europa.eu.int/comm/european_group_ethics/avis_old_en.htm. Accessed on 14 December 2000.

European Commission Secretariat-General. 1998. "Press Release." Brussels, 23 November. Available at: www.europa.eu.int/comm/sg/sgc/ethics/eu/opinions.htm. Accessed on 7 January 1999.

European Parliament. 2000. "Resolution on Human Cloning." 7 September. Available at: www.europarl.eu.int/dg3/sdp/journ/en/nj000907_en1.htm. Accessed on 22 September 2000.

Fertility Clinic Success Rate and Certification Act of 1992. 1992. *U.S. Statutes at Large* 106 P.L. 3146–52.

Fletcher, John C. 2000a. "Deliberating Incrementally on Human Pluripotential Stem Cell Research." In *Ethical Issues in Human Stem Cell Research. Volume II: Commissioned Papers*, by National Bioethics Advisory Commission, E1–E50. Rockville, MD: National Bioethics Advisory Commission.

Food and Drug Administration et al. v. Brown & Williamson Corp. et al. 529 US 120 (2000).

Food and Drug Law Institute. 1998. *An Analytical Legislative History of FDAMA*. Washington, DC: Food and Drug Law Institute.

Forbes v. Napolitano (9th Cir.); No. 99-D.C. No. CF-96 (29 December 2000).

Fox, William F., Jr. 1997. *Understanding Administrative Law*. 3d ed. New York: Matthew Bender.

Frankel, Mark S. 2000. "In Search of Stem Cell Policy." *Science* 287: 1397.

Frankel, Mark S., and Audrey R. Chapman. 2000. *Human Inheritable Genetic Modifications: Assessing Scientific, Ethical, Religious, and Policy Issues*. Washington, DC: American Association for the Advancement of Science.

———. 2001. "Facing Inheritable Genetic Modifications." *Science* 292: 1303.

Garcia, Jairo E. 1998. "Profiling Assisted Reproductive Technology: The Society for Assisted Reproductive Technology Registry and the Rising Costs of Assisted Reproductive Technology." *Fertility and Sterility* 69, no. 4: 624–26.

Geron Ethics Advisory Board. 1999. "Research with Human Embryonic Stem Cells: Ethical Considerations." *Hastings Center Report* 29, no. 2: 31–36.

Gianelli, Diane M. 1994. "Embryo Research Could Help Many, But Is It Ethical?" *American Medical News* 37, no. 9: 1.

Grayned v. Rockford, 408 US 104 (1972).

Greely, Henry T. 1998. "Banning 'Human Cloning': A Study in the Difficulties of Defining Science." *Southern California Interdisciplinary Law Journal* 8, no. 1: 131–52.

Grubb, Andrew. 2001. "Background Paper on 'Regulating Reprogenetics in the United Kingdom.'" Garrison, NY: The Hastings Center. Photocopy.

Hall, Stephen S. 2000. "The Recycled Generation." *New York Times Magazine*, 30 January, 30.

Health Canada. Policy and Consultation Branch (Special Projects Division). 2000. "Reproductive and Genetic Technologies Workbook." Ottawa: Health Canada.

Hubel, David H., Arthur Kornberg, Joshua Lederberg, Leon M. Lederman, Ferid Murad, Marshall Nisenberg, George Palade, Richard J. Roberts, and others. 1999. "Stem Cell Letter to the President of the United States and Members of the United States Congress." 5 March. Available at: www.faseb.org/ascb/pubpol/stemcelltr. htm. Accessed on 5 March 1999.

Human Genetics Commission. 2000. "About HCD: Origin and Role." Available at: www.hgc.gov.uk/about_origin.htm. Accessed 30 January 2001.

Human Genome Organisation. 1996. "Statement on Research." HUGO Ethical, Legal and Social Issues Committee Report to HUGO Council, 21 March. Available at: www.gene.ucl.ac.uk/hugo/conduct.htm. Accessed on 7 April 1997.

Human Genome Organisation Ethics Committee. 1999. "Statement on Cloning." *Eubois Journal of Asian and International Bioethics* 9: 70. Available at: www.biol. tsukuba.ac.jp/~macer/hugoclone.html. Accessed on 3 April 2001.

Human Reproduction. 1991. "German Embryo Protection Act (October 24th, 1990): Gesetz zum Schutz von Embryonen." *Human Reproduction* 6, no. 4: 605–06.

Iglesias, Teresa. 1990. *IVF and Justice*. London: Linacre Center for Health Care Ethics.

Industry Canada. 1998. "Federal Government Releases New Biotechnology Strategy." Available at: strategis.ic.gc.ca/SSG/bh00228e.html. Accessed on 8 February 2001.

Institute of Government and Public Affairs. 2001. *The Challenges of Human Cloning for Public Policy in Illinois*. Urbana-Champaign: Institute of Government and Public Affairs, University of Illinois, February.

International Digest of Health Legislation. 1991. "Human Fertilisation and Embryology Act 1990." *International Digest of Health Legislation* 42, no. 1: 69–85.

———. 1997a. "Argentina. Decree No. 200 of 7 March 1997. (3 pp.) Arg. 97.l." *International Digest of Health Legislation* 48, no. 3/4: 353–54.

———. 1997b. "Decree No. 97-613 of 27 May 1997 on studies conducted on human embryos in vitro, and amending the Public Health Code (Second Part: Decrees made after consulting the Conseil d'Etat). (Journal officiel de la République Française, Lois et Decrets, 1 June 1997, No. 126, pp. 8623–8624). Fr.97.60." *International Digest of Health Legislation* 48, no. 3/4: 355–57.

———. 1997c. "European Parliament Adopts Resolution on Cloning." *International Digest of Health Legislation* 48, no. 3/4: 440–41.

———. 1998. "Final Declaration Adopted by the Second Summit of the Council of Europe (Strasbourg, 10–11 October 1997)." *International Digest of Health Legislation* 49, no. 2: 416.

———. 1999. "Law No. 35/1988 of 22 November 1988 on Assisted Reproduction Procedures. Boletin Oficial del Estado: 24 November 1988, No. 282, pp. 33373–33378." *International Digest of Health Legislation* 38, no. 4: 782–85.

ISLAT Working Group. 1998. "ART into Science: Regulation of Fertility Techniques." *Science* 281: 651–52.

Israeli Knesset. 1998. "Prohibition of Genetic Intervention Law (Cloning Human Beings and Genetic Modifications of Reproductive Cells), 5759—1998." Jerusalem.

Jabbari, David. 1990. "The Role of Law in Reproductive Medicine: A New Approach." *Journal of Medical Ethics* 16, no. 1: 35–40.

Jaenisch, Rudolf, and Ian Wilmut. 2001. "Don't Clone Humans!" *Science* 291: 2552.

Jane L. v. Bangerter, 61 F3d 1493 (10th Cir.), reversed on other grounds as *Leavitt v. Jane L.*, 518 US 137 (1996).

Johnson v. Calvert, 851 P2d 776 (1993).

Johnson, Dirk. 1998. "Eccentric's Hubris Sets Off Global Frenzy over Cloning." *New York Times*, 24 January, A1, A9.

Johnson, George. 1997. "Ethical Fears Aside, Science Plunges On." *New York Times*, 7 December, A16.

Jones, Howard W., Jr., and Jean Cohen, eds. 1999. "IFFS Surveillance 98." *Fertility and Sterility* 71, no. 5 (Suppl 2).

———, eds. 2001. "IFFS Surveillance 01." *Fertility and Sterility* 76, no. 5 (Suppl 2).

Kaiser, Jocelyn. 2001. "FDA to Release Data on Gene Therapy Trials." *Science* 291: 572–73.

Kass, Leon R. 1997. "The Wisdom of Repugnance." *New Republic*, 2 June, 17–26.

Kessler, David A., Jay P. Siegel, Philip D. Noguchi, Kathryn C. Zoon, Karyn L. Feiden, and Janet Woodcock. 1993. "Regulation of Somatic-Cell Therapy and Gene Therapy by the Food and Drug Administration." *New England Journal of Medicine* 329: 1169–73.

Kestenbaum, David. 1998. "Cloning Plan Spawns Ethics Debate." *Science* 279: 315.

Kingdon, John W. 1984. *Agendas, Alternatives, and Public Policies*. Boston: Little, Brown.

Klotzko, Arlene Judith. 1998. "Voices from Roslin: The Creators of Dolly Discuss Science, Ethics, and Social Responsibility." *Cambridge Quarterly of Healthcare Ethics* 7, no. 2: 121–40.

Knoppers, Barta Maria. 1997. "Cloning: An International Comparative Overview." In *Cloning Human Beings: Report and Recommendations of the National Bioethics Advisory Commission, Volume II: Commissioned Papers*, by National Bioethics Advisory Commission, G1–G13. Rockville, MD: National Bioethics Advisory Commission.

Knoppers, Barta Maria, Marie Hirtle, and Kathleen Cranley Glass. 1999. "Commercialization of Genetic Research and Public Policy." *Science* 286: 2277–78.

Kolata, Gina. 1997a. "Little-Known Panel Challenged to Make Quick Cloning Study." *New York Times*, 18 March, B9, B14.

———. 1997b. "Scientists Face Ethical Quandaries in Baby-Making." *New York Times*, 19 August, 1.

——. 1997c. "On Cloning Humans, 'Never' Turns Swiftly into 'Why Not.'" *New York Times*, 2 December, A1, A13.

——. 1998a. *Clone: The Road to Dolly, and the Path Ahead*. New York: W. Morrow & Company.

——. 1998b. "Physicist in Spotlight with Plan for a Clinic to Clone Humans." *New York Times*, 8 January, A12.

——. 2000. "Scientists Report the First Success of Gene Therapy." *New York Times*, 28 April, A1.

——. 2001. "Johns Hopkins Death Brings Halt to U.S.-Funded Human Research." *New York Times*, 23 July, A12.

Lanza, Robert P., Jose B. Cibelli, Catherine Blackwell, Vincent J. Cristofalo, Mary Kay Francis, Gabriela M. Baerlocher, Jennifer Mak, Michael Schertzer, and others. 2000. "Extension of Cell Life-Span and Telomere Length in Animals Cloned from Senescent Somatic Cells." *Science* 288: 665–69.

Lanza, Robert P., Kenneth J. Arrow, Julius Axelrod, David Baltimore, Baruj Benacerraf, Konrad E. Bloch, Nicholas Bloembergen, Herbert C. Brown, and others. 1999. "Science Over Politics." *Science* 283: 1849–50.

Lejeune, Jerome. 1984. "Test Tube Babies Are Babies." In *The Question of In Vitro Fertilization: Studies in Medicine, Law, and Ethics*, edited by Jerome Lejeune and Paul Ramsey, 9. London: Society for the Protection of Unborn Children Educational Trust.

Lenoir, Noelle. 1997. "UNESCO, Genetics, and Human Rights." *Kennedy Institute of Ethics Journal* 7, no. 1: 31–42.

——. 2000. "Europe Confronts the Embryonic Stem Cell Research Challenge." *Science* 287: 1425–30.

Lifchez v. Hartigan, 735 F. Supp. 1361 (N.D. Ill. 1990).

Mack, Connie. 1999. "United States Senator Connie Mack: Biography." Available at www.senate.gov/~mack/bio. Accessed on 28 October 1999.

Maddox, John. 1998. "The Life Sciences, on a Tear." *New York Times*, 21 November, A29.

Malakoff, David. 1999. "Thanks to NIH, R&D Ends Up with 5% Boost." *Science* 286: 1836.

——. 2001. "Memo to Congress: Get Better Advice." *Science* 292: 2229–30.

Malinowski, Michael J. 1999. *Biotechnology: Law, Business, and Regulation*. New York: Aspen Law and Business.

——. 2000. "FDA Regulation of Biotechnology Products for Human Use." In *Encyclopedia of Ethical, Legal, and Policy Issues in Biotechnology*, edited by Thomas J. Murray and Maxwell J. Mehlman, 215–26. New York: John Wiley & Sons.

Margaret S. v. Edwards, 794 F2d 994 (5th Cir. 1986).

Marleau, Diane, Canadian Minister of Health. 1995. "Speaking Notes for the Honourable Diane Marleau, Minister of Health," National Press Theatre, Ottawa, 27 July. Ottawa: Health Canada. Photocopy. Andrea Bonnicksen, private collection, DeKalb, IL.

Marriage of John A. and Luanne H. Buzzanca, In re, 61 Cal. App. 4th 1410 (1998).

Marshall, Eliot. 1996. "Varmus Proposes to Scrap the RAC." *Science* 272: 945.

———. 1997. "Panel Weighs a Law against Cloning." *Science* 276: 1185–86.

———. 1999. "NIH Ethics Office Tapped for a Promotion." *Science* 284: 1749–51.

———. 2000a. "FDA Halts All Gene Therapy Trials at Penn." *Science* 287: 565–66.

———. 2000b. "Harvard's Koski to Lead Human Subjects Office." *Science* 288: 1949.

———. 2000c. "HHS Plans to Overhaul Clinic Research Rules." *Science* 288: 1315–16.

———. 2000d. "The Business of Stem Cells." *Science* 287: 1419–21.

———. 2001. "Panel Reviews Risks of Germ Line Changes." *Science* 294: 2268.

Masood, Ehsan. 1999. "Expert Group to Look at UK Cloning Law." *Nature* 400: 4.

Mauron, A., and J.-M. Thevoz. 1991. "Germ-Line Engineering: A Few European Voices." *Journal of Medicine and Philosophy* 16, no. 6: 649–66.

Mayor, Susan. 2001a. "Ban on Human Reproductive Cloning Demanded." *British Medical Journal* 322, no. 7302: 1566.

———. 2001b. "Commons Votes for Human Embryo Stem Cell Research." *British Medical Journal* 322: 7.

———. 2002. "United Kingdom Grants First Human Embryo Research Licenses." *British Medical Journal* 324: 562.

McCarthy, Charles R. 1995. "Research Policy: General Guidelines." In *Encyclopedia of Bioethics*, rev. ed., edited by Warren Thomas Reich, 4: 2285–90. New York: Macmillan; London: Prentice Hall International.

McCormick, Richard A. 1999. "The Ethical and Religious Challenges of Reproductive Technology." *Cambridge Quarterly of Health Care Ethics* 8, no. 4: 547–56.

McGee, Glenn, and Arthur Caplan. 1999. "The Ethics and Politics of Small Sacrifices in Stem Cell Research." *Kennedy Institute of Ethics Journal* 9, no. 2: 151–58.

McKay, Ron. 2000. "Stem Cells—Hype and Hope." *Nature* 406: 361–64.

McLaren, Anne. 2000. "The Decade of the Sheep." Review of *The Second Creation: The Age of Biological Control by the Scientists That Cloned Dolly*, by Ian Wilmut, Keith Campbell, and Colin Tudge. *Nature* 403: 479–80.

McNamee, Philip I. 2000. "Society for Assisted Reproductive Technology." *ASRM News* 34, no. 1: 6–7.

Merrill, Richard J., and Gail H. Javitt. 2000. "Gene Therapy, Law and FDA Role in Regulation." In *Encyclopedia of Ethical, Legal, and Policy Issues in Biotechnology*, edited by Thomas J. Murray and Maxwell J. Mehlman, 321–35. New York: John Wiley & Sons.

Meyer v. Nebraska, 262 US 390 (1923).

Miller, Henry I. 1997. *Policy Controversy in Biotechnology: An Insider's View*. Austin, TX: R.G. Landes.

Moreno, Jonathan D., and Robert Tanner. 1999. Memorandum to National Bioethics Advisory Commission. "Previous Reviews of the Federal System of Human Subjects Protections," 23 November. Photocopy. Andrea Bonnicksen, private collection, DeKalb, IL.

Munson, R., and L. H. Davis. 1992. "Germ-Line Gene Therapy and the Medical Imperative." *Kennedy Institute of Ethics Journal* 9, no. 2: 137–58.

National Bioethics Advisory Commission. 1997a. *Cloning Human Beings: Report and Recommendations of the National Bioethics Advisory Commission*. Rockville, MD: National Bioethics Advisory Commission, June.

———. 1997b. Transcript of Meeting, Washington, DC. Silver Spring, MD: Eberlin Reporting Service, 13–14 March. Available at: bioethics.georgetown.edu and www.bioethics.gov/transcripts. Accessed on 22 July 2001.

———. 1997c. Transcript of Human Subjects Subcommittee Meeting, Washington, DC. Silver Spring, MD: Eberlin Reporting Service, 13 April. Available at: bioethics.georgetown.edu and www.bioethics.gov/transcripts. Accessed on 22 July 2001.

———. 1997d. Transcript of Meeting, Arlington, VA. Silver Spring, MD: Eberlin Reporting Service, 2 May. Available at: bioethics.georgetown.edu and www.bioethics.gov/transcripts. Accessed on 22 July 2001.

———. 1997e. Transcript of Meeting, Arlington, VA. Silver Spring, MD: Eberlin Reporting Service, 7 June. Available at: bioethics.georgetown.edu and www.bioethics. gov/transcripts. Accessed on 22 July 2001.

———. 1999a. *Ethical Issues in Human Stem Cell Research: Report and Recommendations of the National Bioethics Advisory Commission.* Rockville, MD: National Bioethics Advisory Commission, September.

———. 1999b. Transcript of Meeting, Princeton University, Princeton, NJ. Silver Spring, MD: Eberlin Reporting Service, 2–3 February. Available at: bioethics.georgetown.edu and www.bioethics.gov/transcripts. Accessed on 22 July 2001.

———. 1999c. Transcript of Meeting, Georgetown University, Washington, DC. Silver Spring, MD: Eberlin Reporting Service, 7 May. Available at: bioethics. georgetown.edu and www.bioethics.gov/transcripts. Accessed on 22 July 2001.

———. 2001. "Ethical and Policy Issues in Research." Available at: www.bioethics. gov/nbac. Accessed on 22 July 2001.

National Commission for the Protection of Human Subjects of Biomedical and Behavioral Research. 1995. "The Belmont Report: Ethical Principles and Guidelines for the Protection of Human Subjects of Research." In *Encyclopedia of Bioethics*, rev. ed., edited by Warren Thomas Reich, 5: 2767–73. New York: Macmillan; London: Prentice Hall International.

National Conference of Commissioners on Uniform State Laws. 2000. "Uniform Parentage Act (2000)." Chicago. Available at: www.nccusl.org. Accessed on 22 July 2001.

National Institutes of Health. 1985. "Points to Consider in the Design and Submission of Human Somatic-Cell Gene Therapy Protocols: Working Group on Human Gene Therapy NIH Recombinant DNA Advisory Committee." *Federal Register* 50, no. 160 (19 August): 33463–67.

———. 1990. "Notice of Actions Under the NIH Guidelines for Research Involving Recombinant Molecules." *Federal Register* 55, no. 41 (1 March): 7438–48.

———. 1994. *Final Report of the Human Embryo Research Panel.* Bethesda, MD: National Institutes of Health.

———. 1999. "Draft National Institutes of Health Guidelines for Research Involving Human Pluripotent Stem Cells." *Federal Register* 64, no. 231 (2 December): 67576–79.

National Institutes of Health. Office of the Director. 2001a. "Notice of Criteria for Federal Funding of Research on Existing Human Embryonic Stem Cells and Establishment of NIH Human Embryonic Stem Cell Registry." 7 November. Available at: grants.nih.gov/grants/guide/notice_files/NOT-OD-02-013.html. Accessed on 4 December 2001.

———. 2001b. "Notice of Withdrawal of NIH Guidelines for Research Using Pluripotent Stem Cells (Published August 25, 2000, 65 FR 51976, Corrected November 21, 2000, 65 FR 69951)." 7 November. Available at: grants.nih.gov/grants/guide/notice-files/NOT-OD-02-007.html. Accessed on 4 December 2001.

National Institutes of Health. Office for Protection from Research Risks. 1999a. "International Research—An Abstract." Available at: grants.nih.gov/grants/oprr/humansubjects/assurance/ass-intl.htm. Accessed on 8 December 1999.

———. 1999b. "Report to the Advisory Committee to the Director, NIH, from the Office for Protection from Research Risks Review Panel, June 3, 1999." Available at: www.nih.gov/welcome/director/060399b.htm. Accessed on 10 September 1999.

———. 2000. "National Institutes of Health Guidelines for Research Using Pluripotent Stem Cells; Correction." *Federal Register* 65, no. 225: 69951.

National Institutes of Health. Office of Science and Technology. 1996. "National Bioethics Advisory Commission Charter." Available at: www.nih.gov/nbaccharter.htm. Accessed on 10 February 1997.

National Research Act of 1974. 1974. *U.S. Statutes at Large* 88: 342–54.

Natural Sciences Engineering Research Council of Canada. 2001. "Section 9: Research Involving Human Gametes, Embryos or Foetuses." Available at: www.nserc.ca/programs/ethics/english/sec09.htm. Accessed on 8 February 2001.

Nature. 1998. "Adult Cloning Marches On." *Nature* 394: 303.

———. 1999a. "European Embryology Experts Offer to Advise on Ethics of Cloning." *Nature* 400: 103.

———. 1999b. "Japanese Body Calls for a Ban on Research into Human Cloning." *Nature* 399: 724.

———. 1999c. "U.S. Cancer Society to Fund Stem-Cell Work." *Nature* 402: 713.

———. 2000. "The Cloned Mouse That Roared Is Silenced." *Nature* 405: 268.

———. 2001. "French Council Backs Human Cloning Ban." *Nature* 411: 878–79.

Nature Biotechnology. 2001. "UK Therapeutic Cloning Delayed." *Nature Biotechnology* 19: 192.

New York State Task Force on Life and the Law. 1998. *Assisted Reproductive Technologies: Analysis and Recommendations for Public Policy.* New York: New York Task Force on Life and Law, April.

New York Times. 2001. "Cult Agrees Not to Clone Human in U.S." *New York Times,* 2 July, A11.

Nightingale, Stuart L., Associate Commissioner for Health Affairs, Public Health Service, Food and Drug Administration, Department of Health and Human Services. 1998. Letter to institutional review board chairs, 28 October. Photocopy. Andrea Bonnicksen, private collection, DeKalb, IL.

NIH Revitalization Act of 1993. 1993. *U.S. Statutes at Large* 107: 122–219.

Noguchi, Philip D. 1996. "From Jim to Gene: An Odyssey of Biologics Regulation." *Food and Drug Law Journal* 51: 367–73.

———, Director, Division of Cellular and Gene Therapies, Office of Therapeutics Research and Review, Center for Biologics Evaluation and Research. 1999. Memorandum to Kyle Kenner, National Bioethics Advisory Commission, 5 March. Andrea Bonnicksen, private collection, DeKalb, IL.

Norman, Colin. 1988. "IVF Research Moratorium to End?" *Science* 241: 405–06.

Normile, Dennis. 1998. "Bid for Better Beef Gives Japan a Leg Up on Cattle." *Science* 282: 1975–76.

———. 2000. "Human Cloning Ban Allows Some Research." *Science* 290: 1872.

———. 2001. "Japan Readies Rules That Allow Research." *Science* 293: 775.

Nuffield Council on Bioethics. 1999. *Genetically Modified Crops: The Ethical and Social Issues*. London: Nuffield Foundation.

———. 2000. *Stem Cell Therapy: The Ethical Issues. A Discussion Paper*. London: Nuffield Council on Bioethics.

———. 2001. "About the Council." Available at: www.nuffieldbioethics.org/aboutus/index.asp. Accessed 30 January 2001.

"Nuremberg Code." 1995. In *Encyclopedia of Bioethics*, rev. ed., edited by Warren Thomas Reich, 5: 2763–64. New York: Macmillan; London: Prentice Hall International.

Palmer, Julie Gage, and Robert Cook-Deegan. In press. "National Policies to Oversee Inheritable Genetic Modifications Research." In *Human Genetic Modifications Across Generations: Scientific, Ethical, Religious and Policy Issues*, edited by Audrey Chapman and Mark Frankel. Baltimore, MD: Johns Hopkins University Press.

Parens, Erik, and Eric Juengst. 2001. "Inadvertently Crossing the Germ Line." *Science* 292: 397.

Pence, Gregory E. 1998. *Who's Afraid of Human Cloning?* Lanham, MD: Rowman & Littlefield.

Pennisi, Elizabeth. 1997. "The Lamb That Roared." *Science* 278: 2038–39.

Pennisi, Elizabeth, and Gretchen Vogel. 2000. "Clones: A Hard Act to Follow." *Science* 288: 1722–27.

Pickrell, John. 2001. "Experts Assail Plan to Help Childless Couples." *Science* 291: 2061–63.

Polejaeva, Irina A., Shu-Hung Chen, Todd D. Vaught, Raymond L. Page, June Mullins, Suyapa Ball, Yifan Dai, Jeremy Boone, and others. 2000. "Cloned Pigs Produced by Nuclear Transfer from Adult Somatic Cells." *Nature* 407: 86–90.

President. Executive Order. 1995. "Executive Order 12975 of October 3, 1995: Protection of Human Research Subjects and Creation of a National Bioethics Advisory Commission." *Federal Register* 60, no. 193 (5 October): 52063–65.

———. 2001. "Executive Order 13237: Creation of the President's Council on Bioethics." *Federal Register* 66, no. 231 (30 November): 59849–53.

ProLife Alliance. 2001. "Prolife Alliance Press Release January 26th, 2001." Available at: www.prolife.org.uk. Accessed on 22 March 2001.

Pulley, John L. 2001. "Anonymous Donor Gives $58.5 to Johns Hopkins U for Stem-Cell Research." *Chronicle of Higher Education*, 31 January, 1.

Rabb, Harriet S., General Counsel, Office of the Secretary, Department of Health and Human Services. 1999. "Federal Funding for Research Involving Human Pluripotent Stem Cells." Memorandum to Harold Varmus, Director, National Institutes of Health, 15 January. Photocopy. Andrea Bonnicksen, private collection, DeKalb, IL.

Renard, Jean-Paul, Sylvie Chastant, Patrick Chesne, Christophe Richard, Jacques Marchal, Nathalie Cordonnier, Pascale Chaveatte, and Xavier Vignon. 1999. "Lymphoid Hypoplasia and Somatic Cloning." *Lancet* 353, no. 9163: 1489–91.

Reuters. 1997. "Medical Associations Urge Restraint on Cloning Research." Reuters, 28 February.

———. 2000. "France to Allow Research on Human Embryo." Reuters, 28 November.

Robertson, John A. 1998. "Liberty, Identity, and Human Cloning." *Texas Law Review* 76, no. 6: 1371–1456.

———. 1999. "Two Models of Human Cloning." *Hofstra Law Review* 27, no. 3: 609–38.

Rovner, Julie. 1998. "USA to Think Again about Ban on Human Cloning." *Lancet* 351, no. 9102: 578.

The Royal Society. 2001a. "Whither Cloning." Available at: www.royalsoc.ac.uk/st-pols26.htm. Accessed on 14 January 2001.

———. 2001b. "History of the Royal Society." Available at: www.royalsoc.ac.uk/royalsoc/rshist.htm. Accessed on 30 January 2001.

Scarborough v. United States, 431 US 563 (1997).

Schenker, J.G., and A. Shushan. 1996. "Ethical and Legal Aspects of Assisted Reproduction Practice in Asia." *Human Reproduction* 11, no. 4: 908–11.

Schiermeier, Quirin. 1999. "German Bioethics Inquiry Could Hold Up Essential Rule Changes." *Nature* 402: 331–32.

———. 2001. "Imported Stem Cells Deepen Germany's Ethical Divide." *Nature* 412: 4.

Science. 2000. "No-Show Showdown." *Science* 290: 261.

———. 2001a. "Brain Drain?" *Science* 293: 407.

———. 2001b. "Swiss Stem Cells Frozen." *Science* 292: 2231.

———. 2001c. "Stem Cell Registry Goes Online." *Science* 294: 1423.

———. 2001d. "U.K. Cloning Controvery." *Science* 294: 1635.

Seares, Peter, and Lin Seares. 1997. "Metropolitan Diary." *New York Times*, 12 March, C2.

Seattle Times. 2000. "Pigs Cloned; Hope Raised for Human Transplants." *Seattle Times*, 15 March, A1, A3.

Seelye, Katharine Q. 1997. "GOP Lawmaker Proposes Bill to Ban Human Cloning." *New York Times*, 6 March, A10.

Senate Rules Committee. Office of Senate Floor Analysis. 1997. "Analysis of SB1344." Available at: info.sen.ca.gov/pub/97-98/bill/se..._1344_cfa_19970904_153135_sen_floor.html. Accessed on 20 February 2001.

Shalala, Donna, Secretary of Health and Human Services. 1999. Letter to Jay Dickey, U.S. House, 23 February. Photocopy. Andrea Bonnicksen, private collection, DeKalb, IL.

———. 2000. "Protecting Research Subjects—What Must Be Done?" *New England Journal of Medicine* 343, no. 11: 808–10.

Shamblott, Michael J., Joyce Axelman, Shunping Wang, Elizabeth M. Bugg, John W. Littlefield, Peter J. Donovan, Paul D. Blumenthal, George R. Huggins, and others. 1998. "Derivation of Pluripotent Stem Cells from Cultured Human Primordial Germ Cells." *Proceedings of the National Academy of Sciences* 95, no. 23: 13726–31.

Shapiro, Harold. 1997. "Ethical and Policy Issues of Human Cloning." *Science* 277: 195–96.

———, Chair of National Bioethics Advisory Commission. 1998. Letter to William Clinton, President of the United States, 20 November. Photocopy. Andrea Bonnicksen, private collection, DeKalb, IL.

Shiels, Paul G., Alexander J. Kind, Keith H. S. Campbell, David Waddington, Ian Wilmut, Alan Colman, and Angelika E. Schnieke. 1999. "Analysis of Telomere Lengths in Cloned Sheep." *Nature* 399: 316–17.

Silver, Lee M. 1997. *Remaking Eden: How Genetic Engineering and Cloning Will Transform the American Family*. New York: Avon Books.

Skovmand, Kaare. 2001. "Danish Council Vote 'Yes' to Research into Therapeutic Cloning." *Lancet* 357, no. 9258 (10 March): 780.

Smaglik, Paul. 2000. "Congress Gets Tough with Gene Therapy." *Nature* 403: 583–84.

Smith, Albert L. 2000. "College of American Pathologists and American Society for Reproductive Medicine Accreditation of Assisted Reproductive Technology (ART) Laboratories Is Associated with a Decrease in Take Home Baby Rates of Reporting ART Laboratories." *Fertility and Sterility* 73, no. 1: 173–74.

Smith, Christopher, Jay Dickey, Bob May, Pete Sessions, Rick Hill, Barbara Cubin, Jack Metcalf, Dan Burton, and others, U.S. House. 1999. Letter to Donna Shalala, Secretary of Health and Human Services, 15 March. Photocopy. Andrea Bonnicksen, private collection, DeKalb, IL.

Smith, Trevor. 1999. *Ethics in Medical Research: A Handbook of Good Practice*. New York: Cambridge University Press.

Smith Holston, Sharon, Deputy Commissioner for External Affairs, Food and Drug Administration. 1998. Letter to Sen. Edward M. Kennedy. 105th Cong., 2d sess. *Congressional Record* (10 February), vol. 144, pt. 9: 5562.

Snyderman, Ralph, and Edward W. Holmes. 2000. "Oversight Mechanisms for Clinical Research." *Science* 287: 595–97.

Society for Assisted Reproductive Technology, and The American Society for Reproductive Medicine. 1999. "Assisted Reproductive Technology in the United States: 1996 Results Generated from the American Society for Reproductive Medicine/Society for Assisted Reproductive Technology Registry." *Fertility and Sterility* 71, no. 5: 798–807.

Solter, Davor. 1998. "Dolly Is a Clone—And No Longer Alone." *Nature* 394: 315–16.

Solter, Davor, and John Gearhart. 1999. "Putting Stem Cells to Work." *Science* 283: 1468–70.

Specter, Michael, with Gina Kolata. 1997. "After Decades and Many Missteps, Cloning Success." *New York Times*, 3 March, A1, A8–A9.

Spicer, Carol Mason. 2000. "Federal Oversight and Regulation of Human Subjects Research—An Update." *Kennedy Institute of Ethics Journal* 10, no. 3: 261–64.

Steinberg, Earl P., Patrice M. Holtz, Erin M. Sullivan, and Christina P. Villar. 1998. "Profiling Assisted Reproductive Technology: Outcomes and Quality of Infertility Management." *Fertility and Sterility* 69, no. 4: 617–23.

Stock, Gregory, and John Campbell, eds. 2000. *Engineering the Human Germline: An Exploration of the Science and Ethics of Altering the Genes We Pass to Our Children.* New York: Oxford University Press.

Stolberg, Sheryl Gay. 1999a. "Five Questions for Dr. W. French Anderson." *New York Times*, 12 December, V-4.

———. 1999b. "The Biotech Death of Jesse Gelsinger." *New York Times Magazine*, 28 November, 136–40, 149.

———. 2001a. "Washington Not Alone in Cell Debate." *New York Times*, 23 July, A12.

———. 2001b. "Company Using Cloning to Yield Stem Cells." *New York Times*, 13 July, A13.

Stone, Richard. 2000. "U.K. Backs Use of Embryos, Sets Vote." *Science* 289: 1269–70.

Strong, Carson. 1998. "Cloning and Infertility." *Cambridge Quarterly of Healthcare Ethics* 7, no. 3: 279–93.

Sunstein, Cass R. 1998. "The Constitution and the Clone." In *Clones and Clones: Facts and Fantasies about Human Cloning*, edited by Martha C. Nussbaum and Cass R. Sunstein, 207–20. New York: Norton.

Talbot, Margaret. 2000. "Clone of Silence." *New York Times Magazine*, 16 April, 21–22.

———. 2001. "A Desire to Duplicate." *New York Times Magazine*, 2 April, 40–45, 67–68.

Tarin, Juan J., Joe Conaghan, Robert M. L. Winston, and Alan H. Handyside. 1992. "Human Embryo Biopsy on the 2nd Day after Insemination for Preimplantation Diagnosis." *Fertility and Sterility* 58: 970–76.

Thomson, James A., Joseph Itskovitz-Eldor, Sander S. Shapiro, Michelle A. Waknitz, Jennifer J. Swiergiel, Vivienne S. Marshall, and Jeffrey M. Jones. 1998. "Embryonic Stem Cell Lines Derived from Human Blastocysts." *Science* 282: 1145–47.

Time Magazine, and Cable News Network. 2001. "TIME/CNN Poll." Available at: www.time.com/time/health/printout. Accessed on 15 February 2001.

Toner, Robin. 2001. "The Abortion Debate, Stuck in Time." *New York Times*, 21 January, D1, D18.

Tribe, Lawrence. 1998. "On Not Banning Cloning for the Wrong Reasons." In *Clones and Clones: Facts and Fantasies about Human Cloning*, edited by Martha C. Nussbaum and Cass R. Sunstein, 221–32. New York: Norton.

UNESCO. International Bioethics Committee. 1997. "Universal Declaration on the Human Genome and Human Rights." Available at: www.unesco.org/ibc. Accessed on 23 December 1997.

United Kingdom. Department of Health. 2000. "A Report from the Chief Medical Officer's Expert Group Reviewing the Potential of Developments in Stem Cell Research and Cell Nuclear Replacement to Benefit Human Health." In *Stem Cell Research: Medical Progress—With Responsibility*. London: Department of Health, June.

United Kingdom. Human Fertilisation and Embryology Authority. 2001. "HFEA Update." February. Available at: www.hfea.gov.uk/annrep2000/chapt5.htm. Accessed on 20 May 2001.

United Kingdom. Human Genetics Advisory Committee. 1998a. "Cloning Issues in Reproduction, Science and Medicine." January. Available at: www.dti.gov.uk/hgac/papers/papers-c.htm. Accessed on 23 December 1998.

———. 1998b. "Cloning Issues in Reproduction, Science and Medicine." December. Available at: www.dti.gov.uk/hgac/papers/papers-c.htm. Accessed on 23 December 1998.

U.S. Department of Health, Education and Welfare. Ethics Advisory Board. 1979. *Report and Conclusions: Support of Research Involving Human In Vitro Fertilization and Embryo Transfer.* Washington, DC: U.S. Government Printing Office.

U.S. Department of Health and Human Services. 1999. "HHS Fact Sheet: Protecting Research Subjects." 8 July. Available at: hhs.gov/news/press/1999/pres/990708.html. Accessed on 9 September 1999.

U.S. Department of Health and Human Services. Food and Drug Administration. 1984. "Statement of Policy for Regulating Biotechnology Products." *Federal Register* 49, no. 252 (31 December): 50878–80.

———. 1993. "Application of Current Statutory Authorities to Human Somatic Cell Therapy Products and Gene Therapy Products. Part II. Notice." *Federal Register* 58, no. 197 (14 October): 53248–51.

———. 1997. "A Proposed Approach to the Regulation of Cellular and Tissue-Based Products." *Federal Register* 62, no. 42 (4 March): 9721–22.

———. 1998. "Establishment Registration and Listing for Manufacturers of Human Cellular and Tissue-Based Products. Proposed Rule." *Federal Register* 63, no. 93 (14 May): 26744–55.

———. 1999. "Suitability Determination for Donors of Human Cellular and Tissue-Based Products. Proposed Rule." *Federal Register* 64, no. 189 (30 September): 52696–723.

———. 2001a. "Current Good Tissue Practice for Manufacturers of Human Cellular and Tissue-Based Products; Inspection and Enforcement; Proposed Rule." *Federal Register* 66, no. 5 (8 January): 1508–59.

———. 2001b. "Human Cells, Tissues and Cellular and Tissue-Based Products; Establishment Registration and Listing. Final Rule." *Federal Register* 66, no. 13 (19 January): 5447–69.

U.S. Department of Health and Human Services. Food and Drug Administration. Center for Biologics Evaluation and Research. 1991. "Points to Consider in Human Somatic Cell Therapy and Gene Therapy." Washington, DC: Center for Biologics Evaluation and Research.

———. 1998. "Report to the Biologics Community." Photocopy. Andrea Bonnicksen, private collection, DeKalb, IL.

———. [1999]. "Center for Biologics Evaluation and Research: Mission/Vision." Available at: www.fda.gov/cber/inside/mission.htm. Accessed on 11 June 1999.

U.S. Department of Health and Human Services. Food and Drug Administration. Recombinant DNA Advisory Committee. 1999. "Recombinant DNA and Gene Transfer." Available at: www4.od.nih.gov/oba/aboutrdagt.htm. Accessed on 15 December 1999.

U.S. Department of Health and Human Services, National Science Foundation, U.S. Department of Transportation, Environmental Protection Agency, and others. 1991. "Federal Policy for the Protection of Human Subjects." *Federal Register* 56, no. 117 (18 June): 28001–23.

U.S. House. 1997a. *Draft Legislation Entitled the "Cloning Prohibition Act of 1997." Message from the President of the United States.* 105th Cong., 1st sess. H. Doc. 105–97, 10 June.

———. 1997b. *Human Cloning Research Prohibition Act of 1997.* H.R. 922. 105th Cong., 1st sess. *Congressional Record* (5 March), vol. 143, H765–67. Available at Congressional Record Online: www.access.gpo.gov. Accessed on 7 July 1998.

———. 1997c. *Human Cloning Prohibition Act of 1997.* H.R. 923. 105th Cong., 1st sess. *Congressional Record* (5 March), vol. 143. Available at Congressional Record Online: www.access.gpo.gov. Accessed on 7 July 1998.

———. 2000. *Human Research Subject Protections Act of 2000.* H.R. 4605. 106th Cong., 2d sess. *Congressional Record* (8 June), vol. 146. Available at Congressional Record Online: www.access.gpo.gov. Accessed on 7 July 1998.

———. 2001a. *Human Cloning Prohibition Act of 2001.* H.R. 1644. 107th Cong., 1st sess. *Congressional Record* (26 April). Available at Congressional Record Online: www. access.gpo.gov. Accessed on 7 July 1998.

———. 2001b. *Human Cloning Prohibition Act of 2001.* H.R. 2172. 107th Cong., 1st sess. *Congressional Record* (14 June). Available at Congressional Record Online: www.access.gpo.gov. Accessed on 7 July 1998.

———. 2001c. *Human Cloning Prohibition Act of 2001.* H.R. 2505. 107th Cong., 1st sess. *Congressional Record* (16 July). Available at Congressional Record Online: www. access.gpo.gov. Accessed on 7 July 1998.

U.S. House. Committee on Commerce. Subcommittee on Health and Environment. 1998. *Cloning: Legal, Medical, Ethical, and Social Issues.* Hearing. 12 February. 105th Cong., 2d sess. Serial No. 105-70. Washington, DC: Government Printing Office.

U.S. House. Committee on Energy and Commerce. Subcommittee on Oversight and Investigations. 2001. *Issues Raised by Human Cloning Research.* Hearing. 28 March. 107th Cong., 1st sess. Serial No. 105-70. Washington, DC: Government Printing Office.

U.S. House. Committee on Science. Subcommittee on Technology. 1997a. *Biotechnology and the Ethics of Cloning: How Far Should We Go?* Hearing. 5 March. 105th Cong., 1st sess. Washington, DC: Government Printing Office.

———. 1997b. *Review of the President's Commission's Recommendations on Cloning.* Hearing. 12 June. 105th Cong., 1st sess. Washington, DC: Government Printing Office.

———. 1997c. *Legislative Hearing on the Prohibition of Federal Government Funding of Human Cloning Research.* Hearing No. 32. 22 July. 105th Cong., 1st sess. Washington, DC: Government Printing Office.

———. 1997d. *Report to Accompany H.R. 922: Human Cloning Research Prohibition Act.* 105th Cong., 1st sess. H. Rept. 105-239 (Pt. 1). Washington, DC: Government Printing Office.

U.S. Senate. 1997. *A Bill to Prohibit the Use of Federal Funds for Human Cloning Research*. S. 368. 105th Cong., 1st sess. *Congressional Record* (27 February), vol. 143, no. 23: S1734–35.

———. 1998a. *Human Cloning Prohibition Act of 1998*. S. 1574. 105th Cong., 2d sess. *Congressional Record* (27 January), vol. 144, no. 1: S56.

———. 1998b. *Human Cloning Prohibition Act*. S. 1601 (also S. 1599). 105th Cong., 2d sess. *Congressional Record* (3 February), daily ed., vol. 144, no. 5: S330.

———. 1998c. *Prohibition on Cloning of Human Beings Act of 1998*. S. 1611 (also S. 1602). 105th Cong., 2d sess. *Congressional Record* (4 February), daily ed., vol. 144, no. 6: S343.

———. 2000. *Stem Cell Research Act of 2000*. S. 2015. 106th Cong., 2d sess. *Congressional Record* (31 January), daily ed., vol. 144, no. 5: S151.

———. 2001. *Stem Cell Research Act of 2001*. 107th Cong., 1st sess. S. 723. *Congressional Record* (5 April), vol. 147, no. 49: S3553–54.

U.S. Senate. Committee on Appropriations. Subcommittee on Labor, Health and Human Services, and Education, and Related Agencies. 1999. *Stem Cell Research, Hearings, December 2, 1998, January 12 and 26, 1999*. S. Hrg. 105-939. Special Hearing. 105th Cong., 2d sess. Washington, DC: Government Printing Office.

———. 2000a. *Stem Cell Research, Part 2, Hearing, November 4, 1999*. S. Hrg. 106-413. 106th Cong., 1st sess. Washington, DC: Government Printing Office.

———. 2000b. *Stem Cell Research, Part 3, Hearings, April 26, September 7, and September 14, 2000*. Special Hearing. 106th Cong., 2d sess. Washington, DC: Government Printing Office.

U.S. Senate. Committee on Labor and Human Resources. Subcommittee on Public Health and Safety. 1997a. *Scientific Discoveries in Cloning: Challenges for Public Policy*. 12 March. S. Hrg. 105-22. 105th Cong., 1st sess. Washington, DC: Government Printing Office.

———. 1997b. *Ethics and Theology: A Continuation of the National Discussion on Human Cloning*. 17 June. S. Hrg. 105-123. 105th Cong., 1st sess. Washington, DC: Government Printing Office.

———. 1997c. *Food and Drug Administration Modernization and Accountability Act of 1997: Report Together with Additional and Minority Views*. 105th Cong., 1st sess. S. Rept. 105-43. Washington, DC: Government Printing Office.

Varmus, Harold E. 2000. "The Challenge of Making Laws on the Shifting Terrain of Science." *Journal of Law, Medicine & Ethics* 28, no. 4: 46–53.

The Vatican. 1987. "Instruction on Respect for Human Life in Its Origin and on the Dignity of Procreation: Replies to Certain Questions of the Day." Doctrinal Statement of the Vatican. Rome, 10 March.

Voelker, Rebecca. 1997. "Opposition to Human Cloning." *Journal of the American Medical Association* 277, no. 14: 1105.

Vogel, Gretchen. 2001a. "British Parliament Approves New Rules." *Science* 291: 23.

———. 2001b. "Cloning: Could Humans Be Next?" *Science* 291: 808–09.

———. 2001c. "Infant Monkey Carries Jellyfish Gene." *Science* 291: 226.

de Wachter, M. A. M. 1997. "The European Convention on Bioethics." *Hastings Center Report* 27, no. 1: 13–23.

Wade, Nicholas. 1998a. "Scientists Cultivate Cells at Root of Human Life." *New York Times*, 6 November, A1.

———. 1998b. "Immortality, of a Sort, Beckons to Biologists." *New York Times*, 17 November, D1.

———. 1999. "In the Ethics Storm on Human Embryo Research." *New York Times*, 28 September, D1.

Wadman, Meredith. 1999. "Charity Cools on Stem Cells After Boycott by Catholics." *Nature* 400: 493.

———. 2000. "NIH Under Fire Over Gene-Therapy Trials." *Nature* 403: 237.

Wakayama, T., A. C. F. Perry, M. Zuccotti, K. R. Johnson, and R. Yanagimachi. 1998. "Full-Term Development of Mice from Enucleated Oocytes Injected with Cumulus Cell Nuclei." *Nature* 394: 369–74.

Walker, Jack L. 1969. "The Diffusion of Innovations among the American States." *American Political Science Review* 58: 880–99.

Walters, LeRoy. 1998. "Readings on Human Reproduction: Introduction." In *Source Book in Bioethics: A Documentary History*, edited by Albert R. Jonsen, Robert M. Veatch, and LeRoy Walters, 337–40. Washington, DC: Georgetown University Press.

Warden, John. 1990. "Lords Approve Embryo Research." *British Medical Journal* 300, no. 6722: 416.

Warnock, Mary. 1985. *A Question of Life: The Warnock Report of Human Fertilisation and Embryology*. Oxford: Basil Blackwell.

Washington Fax. 2001a. "Frist Principles on Human Stem Cell Research: Statement by Sen. Frist, R-TN, July 18, 2001." Available at: www.washingtonfax.com/1/docs/bioethics/stemcell/principles.html. Accessed on 20 July 2001.

———. 2001b. "University of Georgia Researchers Announce Cloning Efficiency Breakthrough." *Washington Fax*, 5 July.

Weiss, Rick. 2001. "Nobel Laureates Back Stem Cell Research." *Washington Post*, 2 February, A2.

Williams, Peter C. 1996. "Ethical Principles in Federal Regulations: The Case of Children and Research Risks." *Journal of Medicine and Philosophy* 21, no. 2: 169–86.

Wilmut, Ian, Keith Campbell, and Colin Tudge. 2000. *The Second Creation: Dolly and the Age of Biological Control*. New York: Farrar, Straus and Giroux.

Wilmut, I. M., A. E. Schnieke, J. McWhir, A. J. Kind, and K. H. S. Campbell. 1997. "Viable Offspring Derived from Fetal and Adult Mammalian Cells." *Nature* 385: 810–13.

World Health Organization. 1998a. "Implementation of Resolutions and Decisions. Report by the Director-General." Fifty-first World Health Assembly, A51/6 Add.1, Provisional agenda item 20. Geneva, 8 April.

———. 1998b. "Ethical, Scientific and Social Implications of Cloning in Human Health." Fifty-first World Health Assembly, WHA 51.10, Agenda item 20. Geneva, 16 May.

———. 1999. "Cloning in Human Health. Report by the Secretariat." Fifty-second World Health Assembly, A52/12, Agenda item 13. Geneva, 1 April.

———. 2000. "Cloning in Human Health. Report by the Director General." Fifty-third World Health Assembly, A53/15, Provisional agenda item 12.12. Geneva, 10 May.

Ye, Xuehai, Guang Ping Gao, Carol Pabin, Steven E. Raper, and James M. Wilson. 1998. "Evaluating the Potential of Germ Line Transmission after Intravenous Administration of Recombinant Adenovirus in the C3H Mouse." *Human Gene Therapy* 9: 2135–42.

Young, Alison Harvison. 1998. "New Reproductive Technologies in Canada and the United States: Same Problems, Different Discourses." *Temple International and Comparative Law Journal* 12, no. 1: 43–85.

Zanjani, Esmail D., and W. French Anderson. 1999. "Prospects for in Utero Human Gene Therapy." *Science* 285: 2084–88.

Zimmerman, B. K. 1991. "Human Germ-Line Therapy: The Case for Its Development and Use." *Journal of Medicine and Philosophy* 16: 593–612.

Zoon, Kathryn C. 1999. Remarks at meeting of Recombinant DNA Advisory Committee, Food and Drug Administration, Washington, DC, 9–10 December. Photocopy. Andrea Bonnicksen, private collection, DeKalb, IL.

———, Director of Center for Biologics Evaluation and Research, U.S. Food and Drug Administration. 2001. Letter to Sponsors/Researchers—Human Cells Used in Therapy Involving the Transfer of Genetic Material By Means Other Than the Union of Gamete Nuclei. 6 July. Available at: www.fda.gov/cber/ltr/cytotrans070601.htm. Accessed 11 July 2001.

INDEX